BEFORE I SLEEP

To a great M1
PBL group
4/2/06

Bill Witlen

BEFORE I SLEEP

A Doctor on Call

a novel

by

William C. Waters III, MD

ACKNOWLEDGEMENTS: The author expresses his deepest
appreciation for the work of the Logikon Associate Publisher,
Elizabeth McEntire, for the photography and concept of the cover
and for endless other invaluable contributions; to the Medical
Librarian Sharon Leslie, for her editorial analysis; and to Brian
Shively, for his creativity and expertise in cover design.

ISBN 0-9771288-0-6

LCCN 2005906887

Manufactured and Printed in the United States of America by
Lightning Source, Inc., Lavergne, Tennessee

"It is best to take each day at a time, on its own merits. Do your best, do not worry what came before or after. Thus each day becomes, as it were, an air-tight room."

--Sir William Osler

"But I have promises to keep
And miles to go before I sleep
And miles to go before I sleep."

--Robert Frost

To Sarah Ann,
who pretended
to be having
as much fun
as I

FOREWORD

Which is it: You do well what you like? Or you like what you do well? Either way you probably wanted to make a living doing something that's fun.

But if you look at the statistics, most people missed out.   There were a lot of courses in the curriculum but none of them was named *Self 101*, and so they blundered into something and there they are.

People who disliked medicine and ended up in it are the most miserable of all. They are swimming up a waterfall.

But anybody who actually *liked* medicine and then went into it has a secret daily treasure that he won't even tell anybody about. He doesn't need to. Everybody knows.

This person is a strange breed. And his day is stranger. If you looked at one of those days you might think there is too much excitement, anger, pity, warmth, anguish, intellectual thrill, frustration, joy, and boredom for just 24 hours. Maybe.

Anyway, John Galen, MD, is one of those people. And this is one of his days.

-- William Waters

TRACTION, TRACTORS

Hard to keep my feet together because the snow seems a little heavy . . . which is not like Buddy's Run at all, maybe it'll dry up further down but on the other hand snow at Steamboat Springs is usually lighter and fluffier up here on top . . . the beep beep beep is coming from that snow cat and the yellow light is blinking.

But it's not the snow cat....

It's the *beeper*.

The beeper has a display window: CALL DR BASEMORE 1-912-932-8877 /SOUTHWEST MEDICAL CENTER/ URGENT/ PATIENT CRITICALLY INJURED/ TRACTOR ACCIDENT/ SHOCK /RENAL FAILURE/NEEDS HELICOPTER TRANSFER.

Tractor? Kidney failure? Why me? I'm a skier. But the clock says 5:30 a.m. It also says You're a Doctor. An internist. A nephrologist. It's Thursday.

And you're On Call.

Lloyd Basemore, MD, has a gravelly voice and a matter-of-fact tone but you can tell from the breathy sound that his vocal cords are tight. He has decided not to bother with too many grammatical niceties.

"Right under the wheel before he knew anything. German DDM32, diesel, sumbitch weighs six tons. Brought him to the ER about dark, back of a goddam Chivvy pickup.

1

We been hanging in here all night, me and my partner and half the nurses in the hospital. Lower rib cage and upper abdomen. Not exactly a flail chest but close. No blood pressure of course, pumped in three units of Plasmanate before we got a beep on the Doppler, then five bags of blood before we got 80 systolic."

Bazemore's description is not a model of organization but he *is* delivering the data. "Twenty-three years old, by God, lives up here just outside Bullhitch, belly's rigid, gases not too hot even on six liters. No urine to speak of, Just about 100 cc of bloody stuff through the Foley all night. Electrolytes are naturally all screwed up.

"Doctor, I'm saying we got problems with this here boy. To be plain, sir, we're in deep shit."

"I'm getting the picture, Dr. Bazemore. I already put in a call to the helicopter people. What we need to know, where can they land? They say there's no pad down there." It occurs to me I'm not setting any prose standards either.

"Hell, there's a great big empty field across from the hospital. Fellow had this land, used to put on country fairs. Went broke. Nice guy. Manages apartments. Doctor, you could land a goddam Apache on the sumbitch and not blow any dust in the street."

"OK. I'll alert the crew and get our folks on standby here. As you know I just do internal medicine and kidney disease. But I'll get everybody we need and we'll do our damnedest. What's the patient's name?"

"Treadway. Jimmy Treadway. Good boy. Nice family. All solid church people. But I'll have to warn you."

2

"Yes?"

"There's an army of them."

"That's OK. I just hope one thing, Dr. Bazemore."

"What's that?"

"This army of church people -- have they built up some credit with the Man?

TO THE HOSPITAL

There's a special thing about the deserted dark of the streets just before dawn: it's a little monastic, privately rewarding. Of course there are the night people, just getting to bed . . . Sinatra and the tuxedo crowd, the rock set and their neon addiction, the yuppies and their Pinot Grigio, the jazz folks and their blue smoke curtains. There are the boat people and the street people. And then there are we: the dawn people: I and a few select others, chosen by circumstances to crank up the world.

Like the construction people. The car ahead, waiting at the stop light, is full of heads with jutting baseball bills, soon to be exchanged for hard hats. The heads bob and laugh, perhaps shedding trivia in preparation for a relentless day. Each one, it seems, is eminently his own man. He is sought, wanted. He has a value, measured in dollars per unit of time, so that, unlike me, he need not reestablish his worth day after day. If he is a painter, he will -- later -- assuage the deadly damage that boredom does to his spirit with spirits of another kind; his liver will meekly bear the injury, since injury of any sort, like matter, is never dissipated, only shifted to another place. The bulldozer operator is not in the car; he is elite.   He will arrive later, alone, smoking, surveying the battle arena to which he has at last condescended to come. He will not laugh like the others.   He will shed his jacket, mount his frowning monster, throw down the smoldering cigarette, and move small hills in two hours without a change of expression.   His injuries he has shifted to the earth.   He can now go on, free for a time.

Soon I will pass by the nearby construction site, where the crane operator will have already appeared.   He would naturally want to come early, to peer down quietly upon the tangle of girders and crosspieces he has engendered -- privately to view his own Roman Forum.   For, strangely, he will not see it again during his work period: stationed belowdecks, a big man in his cramped cab, out of sight of his labors, he will follow with utter faith the hand signals that guide the enormous steel logs to precise destinations on the screws.   Like the bulldozer impresario, he says little. Tribal magicians are laconic.

And the runners.   They have achieved temporary solitude, have deserted mankind for thirty minutes.   They have even deserted themselves, sheer dumb effort freeing their consciousness from the fearful tedium of self-concern. They look distraught, but only because distress has now been externalized: the soul is emptied of need and hurt and desire -- at the expense of the face.   They pretend not to see me or my car; they are honorific souls by their own decree. I know; I am one of them.   But today is not my day to run.

Now through the series of gates: carefully insert your card into each tiny slot.   Mr. Bonner has done his job as

4

administrator of plant services: even as he sleeps his devilish machinations regiment, robotize, and impede. Periodically some inflamed soul drives through the wooden arm, knocking it to the ground, leaving a splintered stub. On such days, employees in procession gleefully sail through to their appointed parking places, delighted with a twenty-second bonus of freedom.

The offices I share with my partner Elbert Williams, MD (actually we are incorporated now and are technically "associates"), and my son, John, Jr., are on the third floor. Elbert's son Tom, an amateur comedian, says the designation is a natural for a soap opera -- to be called *Suite 350* -- and adds irreverently that the personal lives of the inhabitants are all the material a writer would need. I enter through the back door -- the quintessential escape route every doctor must have -- and note that I have preceded the always early-to-rise receptionist-telephone-monitor-vivacious-public-relations-expert Sandra, a sure indication that I have arrived before 6:30. But she'll be in shortly, turn on the Xerox machine, type up patient lists, have everything in compulsive order so that the day will not bring one of her crippling migraines. Thank God for people who have migraines.

The hospital lobby, connected as it is by a 200-yard breezeway to our office building, is relatively deserted this morning. Good -- maybe I can see all of the eleven patients in the 110 minutes remaining before office hours at 8:30 without a series of conversations with other doctors. Sometimes intriguing, sometimes stultifying, such talks take up time, the internist's only commodity of salable value.

For example, I may run into Joshua Able, general surgeon: "Interesting case I had yesterday, John. Little lady I'd operated on years ago for gallbladder. Lives in a little town called Doolin. Don't know why people from Doolin always keep coming to me. I like to think maybe I've done a good job for some of them. Came in this time with a strangulated hernia -- colon cancer right in the middle of the thing. Tell you the way I handled it, I . . . ."

"Ever heard of Corynebacterium equi?" Manuel Hammer, MD, is an infectious disease expert. "Just had a woman with pulmonary infection due to that weird bug. "Course she was taking immuno-suppressive drugs for her lymphoma, and . . ."

Let's see--even without interruptions that will be ten minutes each: three minutes with the chart, seven minutes with the patient--no, one minute to discuss things with the nurse, six minutes with the patient.

"DOCTOR GALEN, DOCTOR JOHN GALEN, PLEASE CALL 3664."

Not counting the time answering pages.

The ward clerk says, "Three West."

I say, "This is Doctor Galen."

"Yes? Can we help you?"

"You called *me.*"

"Oh. Just a moment." Then distantly: "Did anybody call Dr. Galen?" Pause. "We're paging Jackie, Dr. Galen. Maybe she called you." Background again: "Miss Sullivan, Miss Sullivan, put on your light please, put on your light please."

6

[A long pause. Meanwhile, the overhead system again: "DOCTOR GALEN, DOCTOR JOHN GALEN, CALL 3266, PLEASE."]

"This is Jackie, Dr. Galen. Can you come down here right away?"

"Yes, okay. What's going on?"

"It's a lab test that just came back."

"A lab test? Tell me the result."

"We'd rather you just come down and see it for yourself, if you don't mind."

"Well, I will. Let me understand--just a *lab test*? Must be pretty thrilling."

TAKE TWO ASPIRIN

The call on Ext. 3266 is to report a blood gas determination on Mary Lewis, the lady who came in last night with an aspirin overdose. I'm glad that at least they're willing to give me the result on the telephone. It's not good, but better: pH 7.54, pCO2 27, pO2 96. So her oxygen level is fine. She's still overbreathing, so her blood is still abnormally alkaline. But much less so than last night, and anyway that's characteristic of what she has -- aspirin, or salicylate, poisoning. The salicylate level is better---down from the toxic level of 53 milligrams per 100 milliliters of serum reported originally to the now merely high level of 32. She could have gotten into serious trouble: aspirin in toxic doses can cause fatal acidosis. We treated her with large amounts of intravenous fluids and sodium bicarbonate, we washed out her stomach, we put down activated charcoal to absorb any more of the stuff that was still in the intestinal tract (that's out of date now – studies show washing out the stomach, though impressive to the patient, isn't helpful). Hemodialysis -- running her blood through the artificial kidney -- was considered, but judged unnecessary.

Funny how the whole thing was discovered. Monica Lewis, an attractive, artificially blonde, recently divorced lady in her thirties was being treated for kidney infection, or pyelonephritis, and came back to the emergency room for a routine follow-up urine check last evening. The ER doctor, Carla Kastle, observed her hyperventilating, or overbreathing, as she sat there in her chair. Many doctors probably wouldn't have noticed. But then Goethe said "What one knows, one sees." And Carla knows a lot. Later, the patient explained that she had been feeling poorly, having some pain, running a little fever, and knew that aspirin was good for all that. Two tablets every four hours helped, so she surmised that two every *two* hours would help even more. Eight days later here she was, with twice the level she needed for therapeutic effectiveness -- consigned to the intensive care unit with a couple of intravenous lines and one needle in her radial artery to monitor blood gas levels and acid-base balance. She wasn't feeling great but she was alive. And she was appreciative.

Now, according to the multi-channel auto-analyzer, she is better.

NEARLY TRUE

I think I hear another page as I get into the elevator, but I'll let it ride for now. I've got to find out about that earthshaking, confidential, non-communicable lab test. And before long, the big event will happen -- Jimmy Treadway, the tractor victim, will swoop down on the helicopter pad.

"Good morning, Dr. Galen. How do you think he's doing?" The short, neat, late-forties woman who enters the elevator from the second floor walks up like an old friend and looks up at me with an expression of unmixed expectation. She looks distantly familiar, but I don't know who she is. Worst of all, I have no idea whatsoever who "he" is.

But then I'm a clever sort. "Haven't seen him yet this morning, but I haven't heard anything -- and no news is good news, you know! I'll go by in a little while, let you know if there's any problem."

What if he isn't even in the hospital? What if she's just talking about someone I saw in the office lately?

"Dr. Johns says he can probably take his eye patch off tomorrow if everything goes well," she says. "He sat up twice yesterday."

Whew. "Wonderful what they can do with those big eye operations now. Just like nothing happened."

"Sure is, Dr. Galen. We'll never be able to thank you enough for sending us to Dr. Johns."

"It's always wisest to deal with the best," I comment, sage as ever. Now I'm on safe ground: Bronson Johns is a retinal specialist. Whatever he did was a big deal, ophthalmologically speaking. I'll ask him which of my

9

patients he's got in now, chew him out a little for not notifying me, go by and see the patient. I may even call some of the family members like this lady to give them a little report. Now then of course you understand I haven't exactly been guilty of a lie. I'm just smooth, glossy. Like the sliding board to the big inferno.

I've told our receptionist, Sandra, the migraine-sufferer, that when she gets to the pearly gates and St. Pete whips out the computer readout of all her white lies, she can officially chalk up her transgressions to my account (since it's already loaded):

"No, he's not in right now, Mr. Handelsburg. He's on the other phone, Miss Andersen. He's tied up in the hospital with an emergency, Dr. Richards. He's doing a procedure on a patient, Juanita, or he'd be glad to talk to you about the Medicare situation on Mr. Berryhill. We don't have any new patient openings for three months, Bruce. He <u>will</u> certainly want to talk to you as soon as possible, Mrs. Jacobs."

Sandra shouldn't be the one to pay the price for all those shadings of the truth. Wonder if it's really as bad down there as Rodin suggests on his *Gates of Hell*. Whew, again.

The elevator doors open on the third level just as I remember: I'm supposed to be in the dialysis unit for the bimonthly meeting on the renal failure patients who are on artificial kidney treatments. God. I'll call Sandra, have her explain I'm tied up, arrange to catch up with the conference later. Got to see these hospital patients. Thank you, Sandra. That's another one I owe you. Somehow I'll get you through those gates (I mean the pearly ones).

CODE BLUE

Two steps into the foyer of Three West, four steps from the mystery of the magical lab test, and the speaker goes off, louder and more distinctly than before: "YOUR ATTENTION, PLEASE. WARD 100, ROOM 614. REPEATING, WARD 100, ROOM 614."

Not one of my patients' rooms, at least. But we all have to go. Ward 100 means cardiac arrest. All available doctors, resident physicians, respiratory therapists, a nurse from the cardiac care unit, nurses from the nearest station -- all convene in a rush (more like a mad tumult) at the bedside of the afflicted. Maybe it's a 90-year old stroke victim; maybe it's a 35-year-old man with a heart attack: in either case resuscitation is the order of the moment.

You see, you can't just *die* in a hospital any more. Special arrangements have to be made. If you don't make these arrangements, the disappearance of the pulse or of respiratory effort triggers an automatic signal for massive mobilization. The team compresses the chest (and hence the heart) at 60 times a minute, others insert a tube through the mouth into the windpipe, blow up a balloon so it will stay there, pump on a little bag full of oxygen at 20 times a minute or so. *If you don't start breathing soon they will hook the tube up to a machine which will do it for you. They'll give a lot of drugs to get your heart started again.* Foolish, you say? Not necessarily. Fifteen to twenty percent of such patients will live, leave the hospital, have a reasonably decent existence, at least for a time. A few are saved for what proves

11

to be a valuable lifetime. Most, of course, succumb anyway, despite all efforts.

Maybe the elephants handle it a little better. They have a certain place they go when it's time to die. All the elephants seem to know about this place. When one goes there nobody bothers him. Certainly nobody resuscitates him, presses on his chest, shocks him, sticks needles into him, gets blood gas determinations on him. He can die in serene, if elephantine, splendor. If you want the same consideration in a modern hospital (at least in our state), you have to sign a Living Will which, in effect, says Stop When There's Probably No Use. Or you or your family can tell the doctor you don't want Heroic Measures, you don't want to be hooked up to a machine. If this is reasonable, and of course if the doctor agrees, you become a "No Ward 100," sometimes known as a "No Code." I have thought of getting a No Code sign for myself in case I keel over in a hospital, maybe tape it to my forehead. The elephant burial ground is the only place where one can die -- guaranteed -- undisturbed; the hospital is the only place where -- guaranteed -- you can't.

I race up the stairs, proud of my conditioning and confident that I will be less out of breath at the crowded scene than the young residents and nurses who thoughtlessly neglect their ten miles a week. As usual, I am wrong. Somehow they have arrived ahead of me -- cool, collected, the nurses carefully starched, the residents carefully rumpled (like the hats of 50-mission pilots in World War II). The cardiac fellow (he's in his fifth year post-grad) has made the scene, is at the bedside, is directing operations in a monotone

12

as strategically contrived as the elaborate drawl of pilots who followed the tradition of Chuck Yeager. The objective in both cultures is the same: *See how cool I am. The tougher the situation, the cooler I get. Nothing is too much for me.*

And nothing much is. He knows the cardio-pulmonary algorithm better than the slopes of his wife's body. He calls for lidocaine, then for calcium chloride. He announces that ventricular fibrillation is in effect, tells the nurse from CCU to apply the electrodes, calls for the respiratory therapist to cease compressing the chest, tells everyone to stand back, don't touch the bed, set it at 200 watt-seconds, now SHOCK.

It seems to me that there is always at least one nurse with ample breasts, narrow waist, flaring hips. And she is always the one to apply the current. When she bends and twists and puts the paddles on the chest she converts the *danse macabre* of Ward 100 into a sensuous and distracting ballet. Will the patient now start on his own? Will he regain an effective pulse? Will she go through that manuever again? I'm still out of breath (from the run up the steps, of course). Mr. Allworthy, a 70-year-old man with chronic lung disease and bad coronary arteries, gasps, the rhythm is restored, the floor nurse gets a blood pressure, Mr. Allworthy begins to moan. The ballet is over. And, alas, I was never even needed.

A TESTING TEST

I finally get to 3 South. "OK, Jackie, I'm ready to view the famous lab result."

"Dr Galen, would you just step into the conference room, please?" Jackie is not smiling.

The Conference Room is more like the Frito Room, or the Coke Room – in other words, the Break Room. There are wrappers lying around. No ashtrays anymore, but half-consumed soft drinks on the table, open potato chip packages. Only in here are the compulsively neat nurses able to be sloppy. Everybody has to have a place to kick back. Anyway, Jackie hands me a sheet:

SMITH, HAMILTON   ROOM 327
HIV SCREEN   POSITIVE

Hamilton Smith is a college professor, admitted with pneumonia. Now that I think about it, pneumonia of a peculiar type — scattered infiltrates throughout both lungs. His oxygen level was low and so he is receiving the gas through a small tube in his nose. He is also on antibiotics by vein. But, in view of the new test, he is probably not on the right ones.

"What do we do now, Jackie?"

"I guess treat him."

"Any other test first?"

"Oh, oh, yes of course, I forgot – the Western Blot – for confirmation."

"Exactly. And then what about his treatment?"

"Well, the anti-retroviral drugs."

"After confirmation. But what about the funny pneumonia?"

"Let's see . . .he might have that, that . . . plasma-cell pneumonia that goes along with AIDS."

14

"Right. *Pneumocystis carinii.* And what's the best drug for that?"

"I guess . . . I just don't know."

"OK. We'll need to bronchoscope him to be sure unless a PCR on his sputum turns up positive. I'll call the pulmonary guys. And I'll write the order for the drug – while you look it up, Jackie."

"Yessir."

"And we'll get a Western Blot."

"Yessir."

"And then I'll do the hard part."

"What's that, Dr. Galen?"

"Tell him."

THESE ILLS

Jack Whitcomb, the senior medical student assigned to my service for this month, comes up breathing heavily.

"I've been looking for you, Dr. Galen. Hear you had a Code."

"Well, *they* had a Code. I mostly watched. In other words, I did what we used to *all* do in the old days . . . before external cardiac compression came in."

"When was that, Dr. Galen?" Jack asks, with the look that says Oh God I'm afraid we're going to hear about How It Was Before Television or Telephones or maybe Electricity.

"Only 1962. External cardiac massage was described in the 60's. Before that it was nothing, Or open the chest. Not so long ago, actually."

15

"Well, that was about 18 years before I was born, Dr. Galen."

I start to say, "Oh" but decide against it. "Let's look in on this patient with renal failure and see if we can figure out what to do."

I recall that the referring physician, Dr. Whittle, shook his head when he asked me to see Mrs. Sinclair. "Severe coronary disease, heart failure, advanced emphysema -- and now renal failure. I don't know if it would be humane to subject her to dialysis," he said. "I've followed her for a long time, she's an old friend now. I'm just too close to this situation to decide, John. Take a look and see what you think."

But now I run into an unexpected problem of my own: within a few minutes of talking to Bessie Sinclair, I am also too close to the situation. Bessie, for all her 75 rural years, her massive swelling, her labored breathing, and her whistling oxygen tube, is an authentic charmer.

"Well, Doctor, I'm willing to try anything that might help, even for a little while," she says, in short puffs. "Course I don't want to be no burden to anybody. And I don't want to be a drain on Medicare; so many younger people need it and can use it better than me."

"Well, but here's the main thing, Mrs. Sinclair -- do you want to accept the trouble and discomfort of the artificial kidney?" I ask. "You know it won't help your lungs, your coronary pain -- in fact, you know it might not help at all?"

"If you think it's -- what do they say -- worth a shot?"

"In your case, Miss Bessie, I think it's worth a shot."

16

"I don't understand," Jack Whitcomb says as we leave Bessie's hospital room. "Do you, Dr. Galen?"

"Understand what, Jack?" Jack is intelligent, interested, and like most students gets intimately involved in patients' problems. Like all of them, he seems very young.

"Why Mrs. Sinclair wants to keep hanging on like that. She has bad heart disease. Bad lung disease. And now chronic kidney failure. Yet she just finished giving you what would have to be considered an unequivocal "yes" to chronic dialysis. She has a pretty low-quality life: short of breath all the time, chest pain on and off, and now the threat of uremic poisoning. Why fight it?"

"Well, Jack, I guess hope is about the last thing to go. Hope that the kidney failure will reverse itself or get better. Hope that the coronary disease will let up. Hope that the chronic lung disease will remit for a time. I guess you'd say hope is the only thing the poor lady's got."

"Seems like anything's better than what she's got right now -- even checking out."

"Maybe, but then some pretty cagey people have confessed ignorance on that issue."

"Who's that?"

"Fellow named Shakespeare said it pretty well."

"He did?"

"' . . . that undiscovered country from whose bourne no traveler returns -- puzzles the will, and makes us rather bear those ills we have than to fly to others we know not of.'"

"Guess he had a point, at that."

"Sure. It was good enough to keep a certain Prince of Denmark from doing himself in. Mrs. Sinclair is a country girl, but, like Hamlet, she hasn't seen anybody come back from the other side of the river with any reliable reports. She knows not of those ills because, in her parlance, there ain't nobody who's been there. It's a pretty deep philosophical point, Jack, and not one that you and I are particularly trained to deal with. And her opinion on this is as good as ours. Better. We have to accept it. So, we'll dialyze her on the artificial kidney today."

"I'm glad we don't have her problems. Or Hamlet's either, for that matter."

"But we do, Jack."

"How's that, Dr. Galen?"

"You and I have to go right down to ICU-Blue, and we'll be just like Mrs. Sinclair and just like Hamlet."

"We will?"

"Yes. We'll have to deal with all those ills we have."

LIFE AND DEATH

As we walk into ICU-Blue, the one place in the hospital where all the sickest people are congregated, I decide I need to drop my musings about the habits of elephants and get down to some real work.

Then Jessica, the head nurse, tells me Dr. Jeffrey Owens wants to talk to me..

It's about Sydney Manchester, who, in terms of severity of illness, is unfortunately the current poster-child of the Unit. A 39-year-old commercial real-estate salesman, he was very successful in all his activities but one: riding his new dirt bike. Apparently he confused the throttle and the brake and managed a head-on with a pickup truck at about 49 mph some five days ago. With head injuries, a leg broken in two places, a crushed chest, and closed abdominal trauma, he made it rapidly to the operating room, where he managed to obtain the services of four teams of surgeons at the same time. The general (abdominal) surgeon Dr. Wharton, widely experienced in civilian and military trauma, said his abdomen was the "biggest mess" he had ever seen – lacerated liver, ruptured spleen, bowel disrupted in four places, and massive bleeding everywhere.

Now he has serious malfunction of four organ systems: brain, kidneys, liver, and lungs. He is on total respiratory support, is unconscious, is receiving dialysis every day or so, is jaundiced, and is getting total parental alimentation (food substitutes via a big vein in his chest).

I decide to lighten up the situation a little bit. "Well, Jessica, is anything all right?"

Jessica is distinctly not amused but instead looks sad. "The good news is everything is stable. The bad news is everything is no better." She glances at Jack for his reaction.

I examine Sydney carefully, check all the lines, sit down and review the chart. Jeffrey Owens, the young surgeon who is serving as attending physician, or "captain of the ship," walks up and hands me a note.

"Who's this from, Jeff?"

"The family – wife, sister, mother, and father."

19

I unfold the paper and read the message and think again of the elephants. It is written in a neat script: "Let him go, Doctor, let him go." There are four signatures.

"What do I do now, John?"

"Well, Jeffrey, what do you think?"

"He's critical and may have worse than a 50-50 mortality, but we ought to give him every shot. He has shock kidney, shock liver, shock lung – all of which could possibly recover. There's nothing absolutely irreversible here, but aren't we obligated to follow the family's directions?"

"Yeah, aren't we?" Jack puts in.

"Whoa," I say.

"Whoa?" asks Jeffrey.

"Yeah. To stop life support you need three things – whether you're talking legally, medically, or ethically."

"What, John?"

"One, the patient has to have no reasonable chance of recovery. Two, the family –technically the next of kin – has to authorize discontinuation of all unusual measures. Three, the doctor in charge has to agree and has to get two independent doctors to concur."

"We've only got one criterion out of three," says Jeffrey.

"Right. Want me to go with you to talk to them?"

"Not necessary, John. You're just supposed to take care of the kidney situation. This is my problem, and my thinking is a little clearer now."

"Fine. Let me know if I can help."

DEATH AND LIFE

Walking back to the next patient cubicle, I remember with a start Sydney's opposite number – Karl Preston. Karl was a salesman too. Machine tools. Also very successful. He was brought in with another problem – total occlusion of his basilar artery. Since this is the vessel which supplies the entire back of the brain and brainstem, he was totally paralyzed, comatose, had no respiration, no movement except that from spinal reflexes. The CT and MRI depicted a wipeout. The EEG showed only insignificant flickers. I told the family that the neurologists and I felt there was no hope. We didn't recommend prolonged life support. But they said they would never give up.

Sydney's family wanted to quit and they shouldn't have; Karl's family should have quit and they would not.

Karl remained comatose on the respirator with private-duty nurses for two years before he died of respiratory complications. His total bill, paid largely by a combination of insurance policies, was over two million dollars.

With Sydney . . . we shall see, we shall see.

TO DIE, TO SLEEP

And now Rhonda Sanders. Last night she went to bed not with a loaf of bread, a jug of wine, etc., but with a pint of vodka, a handful of acetaminophen, and five slashes to the forearms. I'm especially worried about her not only because of the nature of her self-offense but because I'm not sure she's been adequately treated. When her husband discovered her in

21

the blood-soaked bedroom and shipped her in by ambulance at 2 a. m. night before last, we moved ahead with all the usual measures. We washed out her stomach, started IVs, obtained blood for transfusion (her blood count was down by half -- hemoglobin 6.5 grams/100 ml instead of the normal 13).

And we put a substance through a nasogastric tube into her stomach -- a chemical called N-acetyl cysteine. This stuff, ordinarily employed in respiratory treatments to loosen up secretions, not long ago was identified as an antidote to acetaminophen. It was discovered to have the unlikely property of preventing accumulation of toxic products as Rhonda's chosen poison is broken down in her body. If one takes an overdose of Tylenol or Anacin 3 or whatever (there are more than 60 brands of acetaminophen sold across the counter, all of which seem to be gaining favor as a means to do away with oneself) then one's body unwisely converts it to breakdown products which give one's liver a big bang, sometimes with fatal results. So you treat the patient with a bunch of the Mucomist, which has plenty of glutathione, and instead of poisonous end-products you get innocent waste materials.

But you have to get the antidote in orally so it will pass directly through the liver. And you must get it in early, before the damage is done.

With Rhonda we had a special problem. We put the medicine through the tube and in an hour she vomited it back up. So, hurriedly, we got a gastroenterologist to use his endoscope (a long flexible fiberoptic snake-like device), to place the feeding tube well down into the jejunum, the second

22

portion of the small intestine. On the way down, he found a duodenal ulcer which the patient (and her doctor, by the way) didn't know about. So we gave the Mucomist and treated her ulcer with intravenous cimetidine (Tagamet).

And started praying that we hadn't missed the critical moment; that we would be early enough; that the liver would be spared.

Now, in Red ICU, Jack and I look at the chart. Her nurse, Lynn, comes over. (The nurses in Red ICU wear red. I keep asking them why not scarlet, looking for a blush. So far, I get only tolerant looks. I should be more watchful about the sexual harassment thing. After all, one of the surgeons got reprimanded recently for using smutty language in front of a female medical student. Meanwhile, the smuttiest of all jokes come from operating room nurses.)

"She's beginning to rouse, Dr. Galen. And she's mad." Lynn is talking as much to Jack as to me. She smiles more when she looks at Jack.

"Oh? Mad at who?"

"At you."

"Why me? Doesn't like the tube, I guess."

"She doesn't like the fact that you saved her life. She really wanted to do herself in."

"Just about made it. Do you have any reports on the liver chemistries yet?"

Lynn hands me a computer printout. The ALT, GGT, LDH, SGPT -- silent monitors of liver injury -- all, amazingly, haven't budged from normal. A rescue, maybe. A little more time will tell.

With IVs hanging from overhead poles and lines draped over her chest from bedside monitors, Ruth lies in her narrow but technologically competent cot appearing drowsy and disgusted. At nearly 70 she still looks good; she even manages to seem rather stately, a neat trick at four-feet-eleven. "How *could* I, Dr. Galen? How could I *do* such a thing? And even then I screwed it up!" She gives me the humorless, jut-jawed, toothy Vassar smile she has always affected; I don't know why, since she went to Smith.

"You didn't fail by much, Rhonda. But you should be okay now."

"Okay, physically, maybe. But socially, pro-fessionally, economically, spiritually -- never. I've taken a bad situation and made it horrible. I've ruined myself." It is true: her situation is deplorable -- a highly educated, cultured person used to the better things finds herself without financial or moral support. Her husband, a former bond executive, has been deprived of his own debonair status by multiple strokes and has, pitifully, resorted to the job of curb boy at a nearby drive-in. At this store, more pitiably, he stumbles and struggles with Monster Dogs and Frosted Oranges and french-fries, wearing his dark suit and tie. He gives ironic meaning to the song about bringing in the clowns. And now, Rhonda perceives she has damaged her own part-time employment status at a local fitness center with this mindless caper. She is probably right.

I examine her and find her lacerations clean, all well approximated by the neat sutures sewn in by the emergency room physician. Her chest is clear: no signs -- yet -- of the

24

dreaded aspiration pneumonia which so frequently complicates attempted suicides. She has made the grade so far.

"Things are much better than you think, Rhonda. I think you'll agree in a day or so."

"Oh, Dr. Galen."

"Yes?"

"I -- left you a note."

"I didn't see it."

"It said -- how much I appreciate all you've done over the years."

"That's nice, Rhonda."

"And it said --"

"Yes?"

"It said that I took only non-prescription drugs. I didn't want you to feel, you know, upset or guilty in any way."

"Thanks again -- for preventing the guilt. But I may as well tell you -- you *didn't* stop the upset part."

"Well," she says, "thanks for that."

Jack and I walk back to the nursing station and the Pharm D candidate comes up, hesitantly looks over our shoulders at the chart and smiles at Lynn and me. These young folks, working on their doctorate in pharmacology, know almost everything about drugs. Too much, we doctors sometimes think, particularly when these whippersnappers call us up and remind us about drug interactions on medications we have ordered. But they, and their advice, are highly valuable.

"I'm Kirk Sutton, Dr. Galen."

"Sure, Kirk, you've helped me keep up with my mistakes before."

"Doctor, I'm just here to learn."

"And teach."

"Thanks. Anyway, you certainly pulled a *coup* in this Sanders case."

"Well, the liver function tests still look good, if that's what you mean, with credit to the Mucomist."

"Yes, but I mean the Tagamet. Using that was a really sharp move."

"I guess you know we found the ulcer by accident."

"I know. But I'm referring of course to the effect of Tagamet in blocking intracellular damage from acetaminophen in the liver through its action in the mitochondrial cytochrome oxidase system."

I chuckle. I try to make it a scholarly chuckle. "We like to kill two birds with one stone when possible. These drugs are expensive."

"This is where I learn," says Kirk. "Thanks."

We move to the hallway to finish rounds.

"That's amazing," says Jack.   I mean about the cimetidine and cytochrome oxidase. Where could I find something on that?"

"It's not in the toxicology books yet." *(Translation: it wasn't in the book they had in the ER night before last.)*

26

"Why not check with Kirk," I go on. "He's probably got the latest reference." *(Translation: I have no idea.)*

"And Jack -- you might as well go ahead and look it up now, get a printout, and we'll discuss it in the office." *(Translation: I need to find out).*

"Great," says Jack. "I'd like to do that, if you don't mind, get on it while it's hot. *(Translation: I haven't had breakfast yet anyway, and they do a good job on egg-on-English-muffin in the cafeteria.)*

As I move past the heart-cath suite, where Dr. Monson and Wendersmith are already beginning to purvey their long, whippy coronary-seeking catheters, I think about suicides and decide they are not what they appear. When people move to shuffle off that impalpable thing which Shakespeare called the mortal coil, it is not so much a decision as a statement. It is above all, it seems to me, not merely an asocial act; it is a highly positive, aggressive attack on others. San Francisco, for example, is a favorite spot to do yourself in. You search for nirvana, are disappointed by the indifference of New York, turned off by the self-indulgence of New Orleans, bored by the dedicated heartlandishness of Kansas City, and so move on to Rainbow's End: the Bay. Alas, even here Elysia does not materialize; there aren't even any fields. You need, of course, the most dramatic possible exit scene -- ah, obviously, the Golden Gate Bridge. That'll show 'em.

But even then these poor souls are not simply abandoning the society that failed them. Over 90 per cent go

27

off the *town* side of the bridge -- facing not the ocean but the *city*, the country, their fellow men.

Take *that*, world.

In this area, women make more attempts and fail more often than men. They are sometimes said to "make gestures." One twenty-year-old, I recall, slashed her wrists (she didn't get all the way through the skin) in the women's lavatory on the main floor of a major university teaching hospital on Sunday afternoon. Everybody, of course, was visiting; she, of course, was rescued. And then there was the recently spurned maiden who responded to her suitor's callousness by taking an overdose of Benadryl, the familiar antihistamine. Nineteen 25-milligram capsules, and she got a nice sleep and a dry mouth. She didn't know, or didn't care, about the concept of the therapeutic index -- the margin between effective dose and dangerous dose, which in this case is very wide indeed. Neither did the U. S. Congressman who poured down twenty-odd Dalmanes after his intraoffice peccadilloes were sprayed across the nation in 36-point type: the stuff was so safe the doctors and nurses didn't even have to support his respiration.

But every experienced health worker knows never to ignore a threat, or even the merest gesture, toward self-destruction. In Metro North hospital every attempt, however desultory, is honored by emergency admission, a constant attendant, immediate psychiatric consultation, and usually eventual transfer to an inpatient facility, voluntary or not. Sad experience has taught us all.

Women choose drugs; men, guns. The former are only 40 per cent effective the first time; the latter, almost always. Two of my friends and patients became their own victims -- one of them on the day after consulting me for a general physical examination. You can be sure I have since scrutinized -- and agonized over -- my failure to recognize the signs during his visit. He had seemed cheerful, talkative, not overly concerned. No sleeplessness, no agitation, no undue fragmentation of thought, no weight loss, no downward gaze. I'd found nothing serious -- a borderline blood pressure, which we arranged to investigate routinely. The next day he was discovered slumped over the wheel of his automobile, a bullet through the heart -- not in some distant and lonely forest bower, but in front of the downtown clinic where he worked. Take that, colleagues. Even now, on repeated looks through the touted retrospectoscope, I can find no clues.

Practically all suicide essayers are depressed, but ordinary depression provides its safeguards: the people are too retarded to take the action needed. Successful life-takers, on the other hand, are often just coming out of the doldrums, have enough vitality to take the fatal step but yet have not shaken off the pall that oppresses them. Thus, anti-depressants, great though they are, may get credit for triggering the deed.

The self-killers frequently do it in springtime. The birds sing, and they curse such mindless exultation. May is here, the flowers bloom, how could people have the gall to be happy? How could they be so insensitive as to flaunt their joy? Perhaps this contrast preserves for them the pith and moment which Hamlet lacked; but unlike him, they do not lose the name of action.

The other did it in his bedroom, carefully and irretrievably placing the .45 in his mouth, with several of his family members downstairs. He'd had some pain problems with his back and neck, and he'd grown disenchanted with the recent interdictions of the federal government in land development; but mainly this gifted man had found, it seemed to me, that his dedication to hour-to-hour perfection was impossibly frustrated by the realities of this life. Most of us doctors do our best: we reach for perfection, but in the full knowledge that we must usually be satisfied with just OK. Occasionally we must face abject failure; then it is convenient to blame someone, something else: the nursing care was inadequate, the state of drug development is still too primitive, the ambulance was slow in coming. My friend Scott blamed himself for every suboptimal outcome, every venture not producing great wealth, every construction near-miss. First in his class, star of the college football team, whiz at the piano, he had newly discovered a virtuosity at the classical guitar and watercolor palette. But this planet, you see, was inhospitable to him.

Later on, at the funeral, they remembered something he'd said in early May. He had cursed the mockingbirds singing outside his window.

SATCHMO

Now -- my worst decision of the day, the one that's been on my shoulder all morning, ruffling my collar, brushing the hairs on my neck the wrong way. I've been putting it off, hoping for an inspiration, or thinking maybe it would go away. But there is no inspiration, and time is running out -- for Thomas Hopper and me.

On the way to the General Medical-Surgical Intensive Care Unit (known affectionately as ICU-Blue) I ponder the circumstance which brought Thomas into the Emergency Room yesterday: a criminal attack. He was already treading a narrow line between survival and medical disaster before some larcenous and violent intruder tried to kill him by pounding on his skull with an iron pipe -- in Thomas' own apartment.

A longstanding chronic dialysis patient, one whose renal failure had required him to undergo artificial kidney treatments three times a week for eight years, Thomas had also developed chronic heart failure. His pump had flagged, one might say, after many years of working against too high a blood pressure load and too much fluid in his system -- a condition not helped, it should be noted, by his tendency to disobey the dietary admonitions of Missy, our dedicated dietitian, and, rather, to stick with the soul food of his native culture.

When first seen in the ER yesterday, Thomas was alert but confused, somewhat agitated, and very short of breath. The breathing trouble was nothing new: he would characteristically take in too much salt and water between dialysis treatments, clouding his lung fields with moisture, only to have it removed by the marvels of hemodialytic technology. But the treatments would take their toll, too:

31

drainage of the fluid left him lifeless, limp. So, shortness of breath alternating with weakness: up, down, up, down. The earnest pleas of doctors, technicians, nurses -- and most of all, Missy -- to control his intake seemed in vain. Not much of a life for Thomas, it seemed.

But there is something special, very special, about Thomas that makes him loved. The man, first of all, is Satchmo incarnate -- Louis Armstrong over again. He plays seven musical instruments, teaches high school music, alternately leads a band and plays bass in a basically jazz-oriented combo. His very conversation is stage-ready: his comments have become classic jargon in the dialysis unit. The vehicle which brings him in for dialysis treatments is the "Glory Bus." Peritoneal dialysis, a technique which he preferred to hemodialysis but which failed him after several years, was nonetheless "mother's milk." His technician, charged with the rather awesome responsibility of putting him on, nursing him along, and taking him off the artificial kidney, is "a wonderful white woman." He describes the extremes of his likes and dislikes in rather lucid terms: Good: "I love that man (woman), I do." Bad: "I just don't know about him (her)."

And now -- the decision. Yesterday afternoon we put Thomas on the artificial kidney to bring his potassium down and to free his lungs, to a degree and for a time, of the fluid. But we had a special problem: the anticoagulant, heparin, which we normally use to prevent clotting in the machine, could be disastrous. For Thomas' brain CT scan showed a collection of blood (called intracerebral hemorrhage).

32

Furthermore, there were several bruised places elsewhere in his brain. If the blood were thinned, further bleeding might occur in that cramped space within the cranium. Even a technique designed to restrict the anticoagulant to the machine and leave Thomas' blood normally coagulable (called "regional heparinization") is imperfect. So we tried the procedure with no anticoagulant at all; the result was three clotted kidney cartridges and little or no effective dialysis procedure.

So now what? Take the chance with low-dose heparin, trying to reverse it all the while? In this brain-wrenching dilemma I consider the ultimate of appeals. Shall I ask The Authority? Shall I drop this seemingly insoluble problem in His lap? Just because He knows more about this than anyone around now? Make Him the court of last resort and inflate His ego? Hell, He's earned His knowledge, let's all use it.

I pick up the phone and punch 0. After 12 rings the operator answers (we've got to get the phone company to do something about that linear system -- they don't even know we're calling till they get to us).

"Operator."

"Please page Dr. John Galen, Jr., for this number."

I hear the call on the overhead. In seconds my phone rings.

"Hello."

"This is Dr. Galen, Jr." Just like he can't wait to help me, whoever I am. Ah, youth.

"Johnny? Dad. Got a problem I'd like to ask you about. Where are you?"

"Two South."

"I'll come there."

"No, I'm finishing up. I'll come where you are. Where's that?"

"I'm headed for ICU-Blue."

"Good. Got to go there anyway. Two minutes."

THE THIRD COMING

A few years ago, when this man, my son, John, Jr., joined us in practice, it was an interesting week. Fresh and shiny-bright from his medical and nephrology training, he was anxious to please but also intent on revealing his deep self-confidence. In Suite 350, with my 6'7" partner Elbert and our headstrong office staff it was clear that a delicate balance was going to be struck.

Since my father had also been a practicing internist, this was the third coming, and everybody wanted it to be good. Exhibiting a casualness that was only partly real, I asked Elbert one day what we would call the new recruit.

"We can't have another John in here," I suggested. "how about just *Boy*? Everybody will know who that is."

"That's demeaning," said Elbert. "Downright derogatory. We're certainly not calling him *Boy*."

"What would you suggest, then?"

"We're calling him *Doctor Boy*."

On his very first day, Doctor Boy supplied a key fact about a new antibiotic, aztreonam, which neither Elbert nor I

34

knew.   Elbert offered up what is probably his highest
encomium:

"Boy knows a few things, eh?"

With a twinkle, John, Jr., commented that "I'm
coming to realize that my main role around here will be to
keep you two up to date."

"Your main role around here, Boy," Elbert responded,
omitting the *Doctor* and with a slight drooping of the lids and
a faint smile, "will be to keep your mouth shut."

Later that morning, on rounds, I took John Jr. with me
to see an incredibly complex, unfortunate patient. At only 33
years of age, this bright computer expert had lived through
Hodgkins' disease, radiation, chemotherapy, ulcer disease,
atypical tuberculosis infection, and surgery for intestinal
obstruction which left him with a short segment of bowel.
Now he was in with an active obstructing ulcer, malnutrition,
and dehydration. He was receiving total parenteral nutrition -
- that is, all of his foodstuffs -- in a liquid form through a
Hickman catheter in a chest vein.

Just this morning, he had "spiked" a fever of 104 and
his blood pressure was falling. Worse, as we came to the
bedside, he had this comment:

"I feel awful. I think I'm going to die."

We examined him and found nothing new. We
reassured him but not ourselves.

"What do you think here?" I asked Dr. Boy as we
stepped out into the hall. If you ask first, then the other
fellow has to answer.

"Sepsis. Maybe the line. Maybe pulmonary, urinary. We'd better move him to ICU, culture him up, change out the line, hit him with triple coverage, support his pressure. May need steroids and pressors."

It occurred to me that he had said it all. "Yep, I agree. Let me call the office and tell them to reschedule my patients another day."

"No, no," said Doctor Boy. "You've got a full schedule and I don't. Let me just handle this."

"Sure you don't mind?"

"No problem. This is routine for me. Matter of fact . . ." he smiled.

"Matter of fact what?"

"More routine than the office would be. This is Br'er Rabbit's briar patch for a new trainee."

He spent six hours with the patient and bailed him out -- for the time being.

But the startling reality that Dr. Boy had arrived came down upon me on his second day as I walked through the coffee shop. He had on the previous day made the rounds of all the nursing stations and introduced himself. A young and unfamiliar nurse with a green scrub suit was next in line.

"You must be new in ICU Green," I commented. I looked at her name tag. "Jeanne Fulbright, that it?"

"That's right." Then she looked at my name tag. "Oh, she said, you must be Dr. Galen's father."

"I've been here twenty years and he's been here two days," I answered. "That's right -- I'm his father."

The son also rises.

As I reach ICU Blue, I find that Thomas makes the choice no easier. Breathing heavily, he looks at me, shakes his head. "Guess I'm goin' to glory, doctor."

"We'll all get there sooner or later, Thomas. But it's not your time yet."

"Doctor?"

"Yes, Thomas?"

And now he makes everything harder still. "I love you, Doctor."

"Dad, what's happening?" asks Doctor Boy, appearing at the nursing station.

"Let me paint you a picture." I fill him in on the problem in detail.

"It's a toughie," I say.

"Yeah, but I bet he'll tolerate a polysulfone kidney with no heparin and no clotting," Dr. Boy says. "I've had them order a few. Want me to set it up?"

"I'd appreciate it."

"No problem."

"Johnny."

"Yes, Dad?"

"Just like that?"

He smiles, the way he often does, with the left side of his mouth more than the right. "Just like that."

WELCOME TO THE CALL SCHEDULE

But Doctor Boy's introduction to private practice had not always been smooth. The morning after his very first night on call, he said he had a couple of things to report.

Number one was about two patients in ICU who very nearly passed away. Elbert pointed out that both of those poor souls had been hanging on for days and had a hopeless outlook. Why, we asked, did you do all those drastic things to keep them going, when they will surely die almost any minute?

"Not on my shift," said Dr. Boy. "I'm new here."

"But what was the other thing?" asked Elbert.

"You know your patient Mrs. Santayana?"

"Sure. About 93 years old."

"Right. I was called to see her in the ER with chest pain."

"Did you admit her?"

"Yes."

"Where is she?"

"Room 232, on telemetry. Didn't need to go to CCU."

"OK, I'll see her this morning," said Elbert. "But how come you didn't put her in the coronary unit?"

"You need to hear the rest of the story."

"You even *look* like Paul Harvey. Is this going to take long?"

"About 40 seconds. OK?"

"Just do it."

"Mrs. Santayana wears a LifeAlert locket around her neck. You know, you just push the button and they come for you."

"Sure.   But the clock's ticking."

"She rolled over on it during the night and the world showed up.   The fire department, the neighbors, and then the EMTs.   They rushed in and threw the covers off."

"So?"

"Mrs. Santayana, you see, has an interesting sleeping habit."

"So far, this has already taken 45 seconds."

"It takes patience to get an adequate history, Dr. Williams.   It seems that Ms. Santayana always sleeps in the nude."

"Oops."

"And when they threw the covers off, that's when she started having chest pain."

NEURO EXAM

Now to the 3-Center nursing station: I've been saving this one for the last.   Better get Jack Whitcomb over -- he shouldn't miss this.   To the extent there is any grandeur in being an internist, this case, the Basil Perlino case, has everything.

Number One, he had a dramatic event, a stroke.

Number Two, it occurred at a spectacular public moment -- during a prolonged and unprecedented standing ovation in East Berlin, where Basil was playing in the first violin section with the Metro Symphony on tour right after the Wall came down.   They had played Beethoven's Ninth, and the Teutonic audience was joyous.

Number Three, he was sent for evaluation to the Zurich Neurological Center -- shades of Virchow and Freud!

Number Four -- Number *Four* -- he was shipped all the way across the Atlantic to me, his regular physician, for final management. The neurologists I called in here at North Metro fawned over him, pontificating about the tiny lacunar infarct which had appeared in the external capsule of the midbrain and prognosticating that he would recover well. Indeed, they pointed out, the motor function in his left leg had returned almost completely, and his left hand seemed to be perfectly free of residua.

Seemed!

Don't they understand that the delicate agility of those fingers cannot be assayed by any of their clumsy tests? Don't they know that the left hand of a violinist has a life of its own? The fiddler's eyes don't even supervise those flying digits; indeed, the eyes are often closed while impulses from deep within forgotten centers of the quiet side of the brain orchestrate the uncanny process of musical prestidigitation!

No, my good colleagues, Basil Perlino must be evaluated, not by the standard neurological examination, not by CT scans, not by MRIs, not by evoked potentials -- no, he must be tested by nothing short of a *violin*.

And you see -- and this is Number *Five* -- I am an amateur violinist, and today I have brought my own. I confess that it is with a certain flourish that I go to the car, bring the case up to the floor, and ask the ladies at the nursing station and the newly arrived student Jack Whitcomb if they want to observe this neurologic test. Naturally they follow me, a trifle agape, into room 312. Basil, himself a little surprised, takes the fiddle from its case, expertly flips it to his shoulder, tunes it by ear, and tells me that it is not a bad student violin.

He then plays this violin as it has never been played. For, you see, Symphonie Espagnole, with its impossible cadenza, has never even been tried on that particular instrument. Neither have the subleties of modulation, the tricky harmonics, the variations of vibrato of this Albeniz tune -- been applied to this particular machine, this fiddle that I played as a child, that I rediscovered after 40 years.

I walk back to the nursing station and write a more literate note than usual. I indicate -- primarily for the neurologists' and Jack's consumption, and this is Number *Six* of the characteristics that make Basil an internist's dream -- that the final test of recovery has now been applied.

And Basil may go home.

Now pick up the student fiddle, take it back to the car, lock it, go to the office, and see the first outpatient.

STUDS

Back in the office, only three minutes after the opening time of 9 a.m., there are already five or six calls.

Before I can get to them, Jack Whitcomb, the student assigned to my service as "ward clerk" for the month, walks past my door waving his newly acquired article from the library. As a senior medical student, he is concerned about his choices for internship next year and has lately been conferring with his faculty advisor on this point. He will visit

41

all over the country, interview training program directors of medical schools in many cities, painstakingly list his options, be fed into a computer, then, in March, wait like a condemned Christian for the "match" to come out. Jack's destiny, indeed his career, may hinge on that unfeeling printout. It sometimes seems to me that they spend all the fourth year getting ready for the fifth.

Indeed, there is no jubilation to equal that of senior medical students after they've gotten their match for a graduate program around the ides of March; they can hardly bring themselves to speak to ordinary mortals. If you're so unfortunate as to have a member of this post-match species -- as Jack will soon be -- in your office for a month, you'll get no work out of them. If you can even find them. I found one, Larry, in March, asleep in the library. I found another, William, in April, asleep in our receptionist's office. They had not been studying late. They had been celebrating.

Fortunately, this psychotic exhilaration of seniorship has its own built-in cure. It comes on the first day on the ward as an intern. I remember it well. I had eight patients on the medical unit, all my own, and I was suddenly responsible for all of them. As I made rounds, the gut-wrenching realization descended like a shroud:

I didn't know diddly-squat.

I devised endless clever maneuvers to pry advice out of residents and attending physicians: "Suppose you had a patient who keeps running fever but the white count is normal . . . ."

42

Jack goes to deposit his back pack of essentials in the closet before taking his place at the small desk reserved for students in the file room. They all have backpacks these days. The women usually wear slacks, which they call pants. Sometimes these women wear ties. During the early seventies -- when the restless celebrants of the sixties had risen to medical school status -- men and women students alike had long hair which they were careful not to wash very often. In fact they didn't wash their skin overmuch in those days, a situation which sometimes prompted pinched noses and sidelong glances from our office staff. In extreme cases Irene, Sandra, or Donna were seen to walk up and down the corridor ceremoniously spraying Safe Scent. But the offending students never seemed to get the message. Or, perhaps more accurately, they were sending a message of their own: Here is what you older, socially unconscious people need to know -- don't you understand we are aping the lower classes in order to promote their cause? We are the new economic avengers; take this little whiff of Woodstock as our talisman.

They were generally oblivious of -- or at least pretended to ignore -- all authority. In the classroom, traditionally a formal place in medical schools, they went still further. They slumped in their chairs, quizzical boredom on their faces, legs extended sufficiently to show their sockless ankles between the denim and the aging sneakers. They waited patiently for the chinks in the lecturer's armor to show, whereupon they could plunge in with a carefully barbed question, designed undoubtedly to unman the teacher and

43

reveal what they had suspected all along -- namely, that here too, even in these revered halls, all is vanity.

The boy with shoulder-length hair and three loops of wooden beads: "What's the point in talking, you know, about rickettsial diseases when the real problem is, like, malaria in the impoverished areas of the world? The people in our own Cabbagetown need money for food, not fancy diagnostic tests for rare diseases."

Or the girl on the second row with no makeup, a loose halter top, no brassiere and not much need for one: "Isn't all this talk about DNA just, like, you know, a device to keep the researchers in business? Don't we instead need research on how to deliver known medical methods to the needy?"

Or the youngster with cut-off jeans and an unravelling garment which may have once been a dress shirt: "Why is all this money being spent on, like, chronic dialysis and transplantation of renal patients when it could be used, I mean, man, for penicillin in Haiti?" (He had forgotten that I, as the teacher, was sufficiently empowered to exact revenge – I made the young man come up before the class and describe the mechanism of action of penicillin and asked his classmates to feel free to ask questions. He was subdued, but not cowed.)

I always felt, maybe because I was one of the potential targets, that this unprecedented social consciousness and this denial of the establishment represented, like, not so much, you know, an awakening of man's finer impulses but something, like, much more earthy and primitive: they were simply asserting a new power, precociously awarded them by

44

the raw fact of population kinetics. We older folks were just outnumbered. Did they represent a new morality or merely a demographic surge generated by nothing more visionary than uncontained post-war copulation? But then, as I say, this was probably defensive thinking.

Anyway, times change and now, like Jack, they usually look like young IBM executives. Their hypertrophied social consciousness and assertive down-dressing seems largely to have evaporated in favor of a cool practicality and Irish Spring. But they continue immune to intimidation by the cloudbank of authority which hangs over them; apparently they inherited from the Me Era a self-assured ability to remain undismayed by father figures like, you know, I guess, yours truly.

In my own training time we were for some reason desperate to succeed, would stay up all night completing menial tasks to impress -- or at least to stay the wrath of -- our superior residents or attending staff. The sixties children, on the other hand, would leave early to go to meetings of the Coalition of the Underrepresented, or protest that they weren't getting enough out of their clinical experience and could do better studying at home. The latest breed, on the other hand, freely explains they have to pick up their auto, or meet their girl (boy)friend, at 4 pm and they'll see me tomorrow. When tomorrow comes they will ask me what happened during the night, have we got any new patients in the hospital, will I tell them about the new admissions. Sometimes I can't contain myself and will unreel, instead, gory stories of the old days, when men were men, when giants walked the earth, when we

45

stayed up all night so we could monitor the assigned patients, have all the lab data available, and present all the excruciating details to the unforgiving senior staff. They nod tolerantly, feigning interest and, to their credit, are polite enough to stifle the yawn.

It should be noted that these students, in the main, are outstanding people. They are bright, motivated, perceptive, compassionate. They are the kind you want to find next to you in the cave after the big bombs have been dropped by both sides. Many could reconstitute society, very possibly better than it is now. Some could make television sets or computers out of the detritus as soon as the radiation had dissipated; and they would know just how long that would be. They are concerned about success but unafraid of breaking a few conventions here and there. The women are largely recovered from the urgent need for boldly demanding their rights and have generally taken to wearing bras again, but this is not to be interpreted as a sign that the ancient mores are back in place. They assume, rather, that female rights are well-established and react only when some obvious transgression of these sacred precepts occurs.

I can think of no better example than Lisa and Elbert. Lisa Jorgensen is a tall, beautiful, willowy, perhaps slightly icy lady who a few years ago was a senior student on my service. Elbert Williams, of course, is my 6'7" physician-partner, a great fellow who is, however, not famous either for reticence or for championing the ERA movement. In retrospect, I think the whole office was waiting for the confrontation. I can still remember most of the conversation.

"What field are you thinking of going into, Lisa?"

"General surgery, I'm pretty sure, Dr. Williams."

"General surgery!   I thought you'd probably choose something like pediatrics."

As Lisa stood in the main corridor of the suite, well within view and earshot of just about everybody, looking like a *Vogue* model with a white coat, one could detect the faintest color spreading over the cheekbones.   "Really?   And why would you think that, Dr. Williams?"

"I don't know. More of a -- woman's field."

"*Woman's field!*   What is a woman's field, Dr. Williams?   You think surgery is too demanding?   It's been repeatedly shown that women have more manual dexterity than men. I guess you'd like all women who go into medicine to stick to the infant group.   Maybe just change diapers on their little patients."

"No, no, I certainly don't think that."

"Or just counsel expentant mothers."

"No, not that, either."

"Oh, good. Then just exactly what do you think, Dr. Williams? It's not too clear to me." The flush was now more definite.

"Oh, I don't think that women should change little patients' diapers or go into pediatrics or go into general surgery either."

"I see. What specialty, in your wisdom, do you think they *should* go into?"

Most of us feared by now that Lisa was set up for the killer punch. She was.

47

"None. Women shouldn't be in medicine. They do much better in the kitchen or bedroom where they belong."

On other occasions during Lisa's month Dr. Williams would spy her about to enter an examining room down the hall. He would rise and dash to open the door for her. On such occasions she would not simply color but develop a full-fledged cherry rubor over her high cheekbones.

"*Doc-tor* Williams, I'm perfectly able to open the door for myself." She managed a sardonic twist at one corner of her comely lips. "But when I need you I'll whistle. I know how to whistle, even though I'm just a girl."

"But then you wouldn't be angry."

"So that's it, you want me angry?"

"Yeah. You're so cute when you're mad."

Lisa, however, true to her breed and to her commitment, was not through.

"Dr. Williams, I know, and we all know" -- she gestured about her-- "that you're being very clever and just putting me on."

"I am?"

"Yes. And someday someone is going to strip away that fake facade of male chauvinist pig."

"They are?"

"Yes. And reveal the real pig beneath." She entered the examining room and closed the door. With a bang. I wonder what the half-dressed patient thought.

So Jack Whitcomb, whose own reactions in this area have not been really tested, bounces confidently into my office and asks what else is new besides the patients we have seen in the hospital..

"Dr. Landers was on last night, admitted Mrs. Andrews with a subarachnoid hemorrhage."

"Oh. Berry aneurysm?" Smart young fellow.

"Presumably. She's forty-one, previously healthy, not hypertensive, and so a berry is likely. But we wouldn't know yet, would we?"

"Why not? Didn't they do an arteriogram?"

Now I've got him. "Jack, would you have done an arteriogram last night?" Perhaps the only great gift of the classic phase of my premedical education was my exposure to Socrates, who taught me the value of the question mark. It was a great discovery when I began teaching medical people. Never answer students' questions with an answer. That makes them the inquisitors and you the prisoner. You answer their questions with *another question*. That means you, little student, should know, and I'm going to find out if you know. This method also wakes them up, transports them to the scene of the action, makes them start thinking. Jack, for example, is now my captive.

"I guess so," he says. "Don't know how else you'd find out. CT scan probably wouldn't show anything but the blood. MRI might show something, but it wouldn't be definitive about whether an aneurysm is there."

Jack is correct so far: the amazing computerized tomographic scan, which reveals the intimate anatomy of the cranial contents, wouldn't necessarily show the pouch-like weakening of a brain artery which has now ruptured. The

49

even more wonderful magnetic resonance imager (which needs no x-rays but depends for its resolving power upon the ability of an electromagnet to line up the hydrogen atoms in the body and then cause them to vibrate) couldn't be relied upon to distinguish the "berry" from surrounding tissue once hemorrhage had occurred. Unless, as Jack apparently doesn't yet know, an MRA (magnetic resonance angiogram) were added to the MRI, yielding a flow study which probably would show the aneurysm. But the gold standard is injection of contrast material, or "dye" into the arteries of the head – then the telltale bulge will appear. On this Jack shows his lack of experience. And I'm having a good time.

"Let's put it this way, Jack. Why would anyone do an arteriogram in the first place?"

"To show the berry."

"Why do you want to show the berry?"

Jack looks flustered and also a trifle impatient. "To -- to find out the cause of the hemorrhage. If it's a berry, so you could operate."

"If it's a berry, *when* would you operate?"

"I guess as soon as possible, so it wouldn't bleed again, and, you know, maybe even kill the patient."

"And when would that be?"

"I -- I -- guess I don't know, Dr. Galen."

And Jack has now arrived at what always has to be the critical turning point for the human intellect. The great moment when the brain scans itself, riffles through the millions of polypeptide and acetylcholine and dopamine microconnections, riffles again, and finds itself wanting. The

50

moment when the personality, determined to present a good facade, decides to recede into humble reticence in the face of undeniable fact. Here I am, it says, on the ground, I'm found wanting, bring in the clowns, maybe next year. Above all, at long last, I'm ready to listen. The brain admits *I don't know*: the quintessential touchstone to learning. When we reach this point, what comes next is magic. The mind has created, then recognized, its own vacuum. It is ready to suck up the answer and store it permanently. Jack has been primed; he will not forget the "pearl" which is presumably about to drop.

"You don't want to do an arteriogram or operate for several days, Jack. Any such manipulation may cause irreversible cerebral spasm and stroke. And you have a little breathing space: when berry aneurysms rebleed, it's generally at 10 to 14 days. You want to keep the patient quiet, control the blood pressure, and wait. So at this point we don't know for sure if it's a berry. And right now, we don't want to find out."

"Should have known that, I suppose. I would if I'd had enough experience," Jack says.

"Yes, well, some people get experience quicker than others. Depends mainly on how carefully they look and listen."

"And how long they've been at it, I guess, " he says.

"You mean how many years?"

"Sure. For example, I certainly would expect to know the answer, like, long before I reach, you know, your age."

LIFELINE

"Karen Coberley is on the line, Dr. G." Natalie's head is protruding at an oblique angle around the corner of the door facing. She seems to think the intercom is too impersonal. And the telephone intraoffice thing never seems to work; or I have never learned how to work it; or I curse whenever she uses it -- all of which are, from Natalie's point of view, good reasons not to use it. Furthermore Natalie is very considerate: she'd rather look in at me before deciding to interrupt. In addition to which it gives her an excuse to keep up with what I'm doing. Presumably if I'm not doing the right thing she will report me to somebody -- maybe Sandra or, God forbid, Donna.

"And so --?"

"Well she's just having a lot of pain in her fistula. Really sore. Had trouble with dialysis yeaterday. Poor flow on the kidney.

"We'd better look at that right away. Where is she?"

"At home."

"Better work her in."

"When?"

"Today."

"I know. What time?"

"Natalie, do I look like the appointment secretary or what?"

"No, sir, you look like the same person as always."

"Natalie, I think you're being facetious. Now that I look at your pixie face I know you're being facetious. Would you please ask Sandra to work Karen in just whenever the

hell you, she, and Karen think it would be nice. And Natalie -
-"

"Yessir." Her grin is causing her eyes to be invisible.

"Don't even tell me when it is. Let it be a surprise."

She puts her hands on her hips. lowers her voice, and pulls a mock frown. "If that's the way you want it, Dr. Galen, that's the way it will be be."

"One other thing, Natalie."

"Yessir?"

"After you have your conference with Donna, try to find something to do, huh? Maybe go and Xerox something, OK?"

"If that will please you, sir."

"Natalie. you know, it's a good thing I don't like obsequious employees." I figure that should stop her, she probably never heard the word on the way to her degrees in business and horticulture.

"True," she says. "You're not the kind of person who would ever countenance a sycophant."

Sometimes it's hard to know just who has been stopped.

But Karen Coberley, I reflect -- as a medical saga -- would stop anyone. I first saw her in consultation 25 years ago; she was 15. The referring physician said she had rheumatic fever and glomerulonephritis at the same time: a murmur, anemia, arthritis, blood and protein in the urine, all discovered following a sore throat --what else?

It was something else, all right. I knew you just don't get both of those diseases at once. Why? No good reason --

after all, they both follow a strep throat, don't they? A person predisposed to one might be expected to be predisposed to the other. But they just don't happen together. I had never seen it. The entire medical literature still contains almost no cases of such a coincidence, and where it does, the diagnosis is suspect.   Karen's problem had to be one disease, one diagnosis -- not two.

But the intellectual excitement that comes with such a flash of discovery -- like the thrill that results from mixing two colorless reagents and seeing them produce a brilliant crimson -- palled. For this high-school girl -- by report lovely, bright, vivacious -- probably had a disease that I dreaded to diagnose.

I walked into the high-ceilinged, elegant, and out-of-date room characteristic of the Jones University Medical Center where I practiced at the time. Karen was sitting up in bed laughing with Susie, a girl friend who was visiting. Her long brunette hair curled down her back. Her dark eyes glistened with amusement and attentiveness.

"You must be Dr. Galen," she said with a wide smile, extending her hand. "I hear you can solve any problem."

"You can hear anything, Karen."

"But you know, I am kind of surprised."

"At what?"

"You're so young. I expected a much older man."

I *was* young -- 32, too young to savor the comment. I still had a crew-cut which had come back in style -- transiently -- at the time. I had a baby-face. I was used to people suggesting I looked too adolescent for the weighty

54

problems I faced. Defensively, I had tried growing a mustache and then a beard, but the abortive attempts had resulted in unconvincing straggles. The comments about youth tapered off with the years, and of course evaporated entirely at precisely that moment when I began to need them.

"A lot of mileage, though, Karen. I keep expecting the wrinkles to all show up one morning, like Dorian Gray."

"Oh, do you like Oscar Wilde?"

"His writing more than his life."

"I agree." Her grin was absolutely invigorating. "You going to cure me up so I can take my exams?"

"When are exams?"

"Next week."

"Are you ready for them?"

She looked at her friend Susie and laughed. She always seemed to be laughing or about to laugh. "Ready to start getting ready -- you know, one night for each exam."

"But then of course you've been studying carefully right along, every night."

"Of course -- let me see, *Mayberry, Leave it to Beaver, Sky King,* then *Father Knows Best*." She looked at Suzie and giggled. "With a few telephone calls in between."

"We'll see about the exams. First, let's go back. Tell me about the last time you felt perfectly well. And what happened after that."

"I think I'll buzz along," said Suzie. "You won't need me for this."

"Come back. Or call me tonight," said Karen. "Maybe Dr. Galen is going to let me out of this firetr -- out of here." She laughed again

MALPRACTICE?

"Dr. Galen." Irene is standing in the doorway. She is large enough to pretty well fill the aperture.

"Irene, I'm going to have to get these assessments out to the Medical Association," I point out, "even if I have to hire somebody to ghostwrite for me. They have to be out by Friday."

"Dr. Galen."

"What, Irene. What-*what*-WHAT."

"Mr. Whisenant called."

"Oh."

"Said he'd be in and out of the office if you want to call him back."

"OK."

If I want to call him back. I'll call him back, all right. Tom Whisenant is a lawyer. But he's a special kind of lawyer. He is retained by the medical liability insurance company to represent the parent firm and its customer, the physician, when any claims are filed. Those are claims that the doctor did something wrong, or didn't do something when he was supposed to, or was negligent. Patients, or rather former patients, are the ones who bring these claims. Mr. Whisenant is undoubtedly calling about a certain patient. For

56

you see, after about 25 years in practice, I am now, for the first time, under suit for malpractice.

It all started -- or started as far as I knew -- one Tuesday night shortly after Mary Alice and I had returned from a trip to San Francisco for a medical meeting. It was about ten o'clock, and I had just gotten home from the hospital after taking care of a late admission, when we heard someone at the front door. Whoever was there didn't use the bell; he didn't even use the door knocker. He pounded on the door with his fist, loudly. I opened the door wide (I can never remember to use the little peephole) to find a plump young man clad in a brown uniform with gold appointments. He had a long legal document in his hand.

"Are you Doctor John William Galen and is this 2480 Alton (he mispronounced the street name) Road?"

"I am and it is."

"Then on behalf of the Superior Court of this county and its citizens I hereby present to you this summons which commands you to appear and answer the charge that you are the proximate cause of injuries to the person of one Abraham Caisson by reason of malpractice . . . ."

I was sure that he took diaphragm aerobics, that he had studied under Demosthenes (he sounded as if he still had the stones in his mouth), and that every soul in the North Metro area had already digested every syllable. Even so, this was better than some of the cases I had heard about, in which the deputy sheriff comes to the office window and goes through the eight-hundred decibel routine in front of all the patients, employees, drug salesmen, and presumably God,.

Then my deputy seemed to relax and smile a little. "Hate to present you with this here token, Doctor, but it seems like this feller needs a little vacation money. Har, har, har."

The stunned feeling settled in, but this benign sensation of merely being shocked was not to remain. Nothing from that point on, it turned out -- *nothing* -- would ever be quite the same. After a patient has sued you, you can hardly think about anything else for months. You go to bed with it on your mind, wake up with it, cogitate over it between patients. You can't imagine you did anything wrong.

Or can you? Then you begin to have self-doubts: he claims I never told him he had serious kidney disease. Could that be true? Of course not --we discusssed it over and over. I made notes of the conversation. Furthermore he is a health worker, a Master of Public Health, and he should know anyway. Wait a minute -- I gave a full dissertation on his disease and how he would have progressive kidney failure and how he would undoubtedly have to go on dialysis or get a transplant between 45-55 years of age -- *to the public courtroom at his divorce trial and he was there listening!* And so was the court reporter! We'll just get those records. But he said I didn't start him on dialysis when I should. Absurd. The next nephrologist he went to didn't start him either--for nearly a year. The suit maintains I should have treated his anemia in 1978. Hell, it's better not to transfuse kidney failure patients 'til you have to, anyway. Furthermore the wonderful drug erythropoeitin, for kidney anemia, wasn't invented then. By the way, he didn't even *have* anemia in

58

1978.   Well, it's all ridiculous.   Or is it?   Am I to be ruined anyway?   Probable headlines:

Prominent Physician Accused of
Negligence by Public Health Expert

Through.   Washed up.   No matter how the case comes out, the headlines will put a lifetime of hard work and careful reputation-building on the rocks in one day.

With every patient you see thereafter you wonder: will this one sue me?   Have I done enough tests to rule out the possibility of missing a diagnosis?   Are my records complete?   Should I screen patients before I see them in the first place?

Can I, indeed, go on?

The malpractice, or professional liability, thing has gotten out of hand.   My state twenty years ago was forty-something in the country in cases filed.   Then it was number four, having passed California in its hyperdrive ascent.   Now it's improving a little again, partly due to tort legislation.   A young neurosurgeon by the name of Henry Oakland -- who by the way has never been sued -- told me last week he just got his annual premium notice: $160,000.   That's $300+ before you get out of bed each morning, and the return on that investment is zero.   As a matter of fact, you can't even get your principal back.

The medical situation, of course, is just part of a national liability crisis: auto insurance prices in Miami are spectacular; some manufacturers of food wrappers had annual insurance costs go from $14,000 one year to $100,000 the next to unobtainable the next; architects have to scramble to get any coverage. It wasn't too surprising that the man sued Sears because his mower was slow starting and he had a heart attack (after all this is America -- pronounced Murraka); what is hard to believe is he won the case and was awarded more than a million dollars.

It occurs to me that the implications of this are serious: paranoia has run amok in our land; the judiciary is acquiring power at a rate never foreseen by those very imaginative creators of the tripartite checks-and-balances system; the habit of turning to Orwell's "big brother" to settle the least dispute is becoming entrenched. Worse, the creative risk-urge of business is being stifled beyond recovery. Why buy new machines if their products create liability more prominent than the ability to recover profits? Why invest in American industry if its tools, already approaching obsolescence, have no serious prospect of replacement? Japan and Germany don't have this problem -- either with obsolescence or unbridled liability -- and they were eating us alive until they developed other difficulties. Confidence, that ethereal everything, evaporates, the stock market swallows dust, our economy and our national well-being progressively decline.

I wondered aloud to a lawyer patient-friend recently about this national trend and he said, Here's the deal: you've just got to have something to replace the deep-rooted American urge to meet, armed with six-guns, on the main street of Dodge at high noon. That is, the opportunity for good old-fashioned open aggression has been submerged by

60

civilization and it has to surface somewhere -- why not the courts?

At any rate, back at my own particular ranch, later information disclosed that my plaintiff is sort of a professional suer. Though a medical professional, he has now gone to a not-very-trendy night law school and spends his time in court as an expert witness to everything from surgical malpractice (he hasn't been in an operating room perhaps ever) to injury cases. He can't take his bar exam because of questions about his character raised by the efforts of the county medical clinic to throw him off the staff (they finally gave up after years of litigation).

Nonetheless the sting is there, though it lessens after six months and after you realize it will be two to five years before this comes to court. Then your lawyer moves for a summary judgement -- i.e., get the judge to declare the whole thing a nuisance case and throw it out. You learn that the judge is inclined to do this, particularly after finding that the statute of limitations had expired on all but the very last visit of the patient. But then the plaintiff's lawyer alleges fraud. *Fraud*! And fraud has no time limitations.

The dulcet-toned administrative assistant answers (lawyers can afford to hire dulcet-toned administrative assistants). "Can I help you, Doctor?"

"Is Mr. Whisenant available?" There's something new in the pit of my stomach.

"Oh, he just left for court. Can I have him call you back? He'll probably check his messages during the recesses."

61

"Yes, please." I want to say *pretty* please. I give her my cell phone number and check to make sure it's charged.

FLUSHES

"Diana Sorensen is in Room Two, Dr. Galen," says Donna in her usual tone, which falls somewhere between managerial and bossy.

Diana, Diana -- God, what a diagnostic problem. She's back now for a follow-up after her last hospitalization about a week ago. Only 23 years old, vivacious and lovely, she's had three bizarre episodes in the last four months. She'd have shortness of breath, a generalized rash, fast heart beat, and low blood pressure, diarrhea, nausea and vomiting. Hospitalized each time, she recovered within forty-eight to seventy-two hours.

The first time I remember well. Dr. Rowe, the emergency room physician, called me to see Diana at about nine p. m. one Tuesday night.

"John, I've got a girl down here with all kinds of symptoms. Flushed, short of breath. Probably hyper-ventilating. But the thing that worries me is her heart rate-- about 160. Don't know if it's PAT or what. Mind looking at her?"

Diana was indeed in distress. She was pink all over. Her eyes were red. She was breathing fast and deep. Her pulse rate varied from 150 to 160 per minute. The EKG

62

showed that her basic rhythm was sinus tachycardia--that is, the normal beat speeded up, as in exercise. Not PAT, or paroxysmal atrial tachycardia, which is absolutely regular. Blood pressure was about normal for a young woman--90/60--but it dropped to 70/60 if her head was elevated on the mechanical stretcher. Blood gases showed she was indeed overventilating. The oxygen level in the blood of her arteries while breathing room air was not low but a little high.

"This came on me all of a sudden this afternoon, Dr. Galen," she said. Her pupils were widely dilated. "Just weak, and short of breath, and nauseated."

"How about this flushing?"

"Oh, I flush all the time. More so lately."

"I bet not like this." Her skin was almost the color of baked lobster.

I asked Diana a lot of questions, of course. Nothing very interesting turned up until I got to this one: "Diana, you say you are menstruating now. Are you by chance using a tampon?"

"Yes, sir."

"Do you always?"

"Yes sir."

"Diana, this may be important: how long has this one been in?"

"Well, it's near the end of my period, and it's not very heavy. So--well, I guess it's been in about 48 hours."

There's a point in the diagnostic investigation of any acutely ill patient when the physician moves from anxious uncertainty to anxious action, and this was it. Diana had

63

provided me with all the data I needed for a presumptive diagnosis of toxic shock syndrome, and so I moved. I completed her examination, removed the tampon, cultured it and the surrounding fluid, ordered blood cultures, started an intravenous line, began rapid infusions of saline, gave a large dose of Solu-medrol, a cortisone derivative, and began penicillin, effective against the Streptococcus, and Vancomycin, an antibiotic with a powerful action against Staphylococcus, even when that notorious bug has developed drug resistance.

The nurses moved, too. After all, this was a young woman their age with a serious, potentially fatal, but treatable disorder. They could "relate" to toxic shock.

Diana was admitted to the hospital and I had her seen by Carlton Lowndes, MD, a very bright and informed infectious disease specialist, who approved of the diagnosis and treatment. She was much improved by the following morning and symptom-free within forty-eight hours. The bacterial cultures of her blood were negative. Of course, in toxic shock syndrome, blood cultures are usually non-revealing. The bad actor is the toxin-producing staph in the vagina, which presumably grows wild and fast in the presence of menstrual blood, especially when an obstructing tampon is in place for a prolonged period. The toxin enters the blood stream, triggers the body's inflammatory cascade, produces the red flush (almost like scarlet fever) and can cause shock, kidney failure, lung failure, even death. But nothing grew from the vaginal material, either, except ordinary bacteria

64

which usually populate that area. Not unusual, either, Carlton pointed out.

The weird thing is that she had two subsequent admissions over the next three months -- with very similar symptoms and findings – even though she had stopped using tampons. In each case she had rash, fast pulse, shortness of breath with a normal chest X-ray. In each case she received antibiotics, IV fluids, and in each case she got well in 48 hours. I called in several consultants--Lowndes again, Tindler, an allergist, Cottingham, a rheumatologist. Horton, the medical resident, saw her. Elbert Williams, my partner, admitted her on one of the occasions. We were all confused.

Then Horton, two years out of medical school, had a brainstorm. He found out she had been taking ibuprofen, an over-the-counter medication for aches and pains, before the third admission. Later, she remembered taking this drug before each of the spells. Horton dived into the library computer, did a search of the medical literature, and turned up one previously reported similar case, in which a woman had two episodes like Diana's after exposure and then re-exposure to ibuprofen. The allergist said he wasn't sure about the relationship to the drug but was afraid to test her and advised that she leave it off permanently. Diana was advised never to take this drug or any in the same family of so-called "non-steroidal anti-inflammatory agents," a group which actually includes aspirin.

Dr. Horton, second-year resident, was the hero. So far.

Today Diana says she feels fine. Actually, it's a little more than that. "I feel absolutely fabulous, Dr. Galen."

I find that I don't feel so fabulous. I'm still worried about the diagnosis, worried she'll have another spell, worried what the outcome will be, since we aren't sure what we're doing. I examine her. The lobster rash is gone completely. But now I find some small spots over her abdomen. They are brownish-reddish, vary in size, are not in sun-exposed areas.

"How long have you had these little freckles, Diana?"

"Oh, a long time. They've been coming the last few years."

Now it's time for old Dr. Galen to have a brainstorm. I stroke a clump of the freckles with my fingernail. Almost instantly there is a reddening in the area, then a hive springs up. There is, in other words, a local lobster effect.

"Wow, that stings and itches," Dr. Galen.

The area is now fiery red. There is a scarlet track everywhere my fingernail touched; I remember this is called "Koebner's sign."

Now my pupils are dilated. I have Donna instruct Diana on collecting a 24-hour urine specimen for histamine, then tell her we'll talk again in a few days. I walk out of the examining room, through the lab, toward the back exit of the suite. Sandra, Cheryl, Donna all look at me and then at each other.

"Are you leaving, Dr. Galen?" Donna still sounds pretty managerial. "We have Mrs. Appleby and Mr. Johnson in examining rooms and Miss Hanson is coming in the door, now."

66

"Yeah. I'm going to the hospital X-ray department. Something important."

"Yes, well, how long do you think, you know, you'll be gone?"

Not long. It doesn't take long to confirm world-shaking discoveries." They look at me again, and then, again, at each other. Then Donna, I notice, looks at the ceiling.

Nothing, it seems, could be less thrilling to the clerks in the X-ray file room than stopping what they are doing and getting me Diana Sorensen's films. What they were doing was planning the weekend. They aren't apparently attuned to shaking the world this morning. Finally, the films are produced and I array them on the ten-plate multi-viewer.

"Steve, I wish you'd look at these with me." The newest addition, whoever he is, to our outstanding staff of MD radiologists at the hospital is usually referred to as "the boy wonder." Steve Wilson, being the latest, carries that appellation. "This is your chance to live up to your reputation as Batman's assistant," I tell him.

He smiles tolerantly and I tell him the story. "All these films have been read as normal over the last few months. But aren't the bones abnormally dense? Isn't there a little bit of sclerosis alternating with areas of rarefaction?"

"I believe you're right," he says. "I'd have to agree that these bones are abnormal. Of course, there's a big differential -- renal failure, osteosclerosis, a long list."

"Right. But she doesn't have any of those," I put in. "Could the list include -- primary systemic mastocytosis?"

67

"Well, yes, it could. Now that you mention it -- these are exactly the changes you'd expect. Let me show these around the department."

Of course, no day is exactly the same after you've had a Eureka moment. Particularly if you've "scooped" some sharp people, like the infectious disease man, the allergist, the whole x-ray department. The Eureka experience dominates the rest of the 24-hour period. On the way back to the office, I think about the bizarre condition we have almost certainly established. Primary systemic mastocytosis is extremely rare. As I remember, not more than 1000 cases have ever been reported. It is a disorder in which "mast cells," a special kind of cell normally restricted to the bone marrow, proliferate in the body. They can lodge in the skin (hence the freckles), multiply in the bone marrow (hence the x-ray changes), the liver, the intestine, the lung. The peculiar thing is that these cells contain granules which, when they disrupt, release histamine and other substances which cause the flushing, low blood pressure and intestinal upset. A lot of things can cause these cells to release their loads of bad humors -- trauma, infection, drugs, even emotional upset. Stroking the mast cells in the skin does it. In Diana's case maybe, just maybe, the ibuprofen triggered the release. Treatment includes blocking agents, like anti-histamines, cimetidine (Tagamet), and a newer agent, cromylyn.

"Don't know why I even bother with X-rays and tests and such," I say as I reenter the back door of the office. "If you're fantastically brilliant you only need to talk to the patients and examine them, write the diagnosis down, start treatment and go home. I may even be able to handle everything over the telephone. Don't even need an office. Reduce the overhead to zero."

Donna is still looking a little long-suffering. "Yes, Dr. Galen, we know. We wonder why we even bother to come in, with you available and all." I think I see her look up at the ceiling again. "Appleby is still in Room 4, Johnson is in Room 5, and Hanson is still in the waiting room."

"OK, Donna, OK."

"And they're all tired of waiting."

"And so are you?"

"Doesn't matter about me. I stay tired." She laughs a little. That's what makes her lovable.

SHADES OF VIENNA

I dial Mr. Henkel back. He has left word simply saying he wants to tell me something. Normally I defer non-urgent calls to later in the day, but any message from the very Austrian Mr. Henkel is a rare thing. While I'm trying to get the number, I remember his first hospital admission, some six years earlier. He had come in with high fever and low blood pressure. In spite of his advanced age of 90, he was a viable fellow and we investigated thoroughly. ERCP (putting a tube down through the stomach into the intestine and squirting dye into the common bile duct) had showed about twelve stones there, even though his gallbladder had been previously removed. We explained that without surgery he would probably have more fever, more shock, and that he might die in the process.

"Doctor," he said. "I'm sure you are giving me your best advice. And furthermore, I'm sure you are correct. But I have lived 90 years and I think I'll just continue doing what I am doing."

Mrs. Henkel answers the phone. She explains he is out in the yard and will return my call shortly. I think back to the second admission, now two years ago. I had been called to the emergency facility of the hospital.

"Don't tell me something has come up you can't handle, Dr. Julie."

"Just wanted you to confirm my diagnosis, Dr. G," she said, with precisely the same glittering smile I had hoped to provoke. Nurse Julie Higgins is widely appreciated as a redeeming visual phenomenon of the Emergency Room at North Metro Hospital. She also has a sense of humor and, unlike a lot of women with her attributes, can actually tell a joke without screwing it up.

She is also a hell of a nurse. "Your Mr. Henkel is a Viennese doll, but I'm worried about him. His vital signs are okay, and I don't see anything fancy on his cardiogram, but they brought him in with chest pain and syncope. At age 92 I guess we have to be concerned." She did something with her mouth and chin which said this is my understatement for the day.

Together we walked back to see him in the Cardiac Room. This is a large chamber where all the appurtenances are available for you to have a heart attack with all its complications in a very fashionable way. Mr. Henkel peered

70

back through his pince-nez from the examining table; in this oyster-shell-white hygienic desert, his already bird-like physique seemed to shrink to the dimensions of a wren.

"I was just getting off the bus, Dr. G, and I had this pain," he said in barely corrupted old-world Austrian-English. He grasped the center of of his chest. "Then I don't remember anything else. Sorry to bother you."

I squeezed his hand and patted his shoulder as Julie said, "He passed out on the street and the ambulance brought him. The emergency techs said he was out cold. No signs of significant trauma, just an abrasion over his right eye."

"How often have you been having this pain, Mr. Henkel?"

"Oh, not too often."

"Once a week? Once a month?"

"Oh, more than that."

"Every day?" I've finally learned that the more guarded a person is about describing the frequency of an event the more frequent it's likely to be.

"Well, maybe several times a day."

"How often do you pass out?"

"Not too often."

"Once a week?"

"Maybe." He tossed his head from side to side as if making a philosophical point during a conversation in an Innsbruck coffee-house.

I examined his heart and lungs. The ribs jutted so prominently I had trouble getting contact between skin and

71

stethoscope. "Mr. Henkel, we need to bring you into the hospital, check some things, and watch you for a day or two."

"Doctor, whatever you say. But if I may, I'd like to ask a question or two." He said *qveshon*.

"Certainly."

"What will you look for?"

"Well, first, we'll want to rule out a heart attack."

"Yes." He said *yayce*.

"And try to get you on the right medication for your angina."

"Yayce."

"And monitor you to see if your heart is having serious rhythm upsets, like maybe even pauses that might account for your fainting."

"Yayce. And, Doctor, what will you do if my heart is having pauses?"

"We might recommend a pacemaker."

"And, Doctor, if I'm having pauses and you put in a pacemaker --"

"Yes, sir?" I can see that Mr. Henkel is following the conversation with no trouble.

"In that case I would have another question." In fact, maybe he's taking the conversation over.

"Yes, sir?"

"I wonder -- with a pacemaker -- then just how would I ever die?"

Julie Higgins was looking at me now. Her high color had gotten higher and she was not controlling a grin.

I squeezed his hand again. "Mr. Henkel, you come into the hospital and we'll just talk about it."

"Good, doctor, That's what I'd like."

Irene buzzes me. "He's on the line now."

"How are you, Mr. Henkel?"

"Fine, Doctor, fine. That's what I wanted to talk to you about. I haven't needed any medical attention. I haven't been to any other doctor. I just wanted you to know that I've been doing well and I still consider myself your patient."

"Sure, Mr. Henkel. Glad to hear from you, but you know I'm available anytime you need me."

"Yayce. Well, I haven't come in for some time and I just wanted to make sure you know that you're the only doctor I ever want to have. You see, I'm concerned that I haven't always done just what you advised in the past."

I laugh. "That's okay, Mr. Henkel, you've done pretty well for yourself anyway. How old are you now?"

"Let's see, Dr. G. I'm 96."

THE MEMO

I find myself rushing through routine tasks, thinking about Diana Sorensen, the young woman with mastocytosis. Finally, I get a break, tell Irene not to bother me with calls for a little while, shut my office door, and dictate a truly eloquent memorandum about Diana. It is addressed to every physician who has seen her, or seen her films, or talked about her. The list includes Dr. Rowe (the ER doctor) Dr. Williams (my partner), Dr. Tindler (the allergist), Dr. Lowndes (the

73

infectious disease man), Dr. Horton (the resident), every radiologist who has seen her films, even an orthopedist who had admitted her with pelvic fractures a year earlier. I even think of sending a copy to Dr. Jan Waldenstrom, the Swedish researcher who has done so much work on the disease, just to show him how smart I am.

The memo recounts the whole story. It tells about stage one, when we thought she had toxic shock; stage two, when we didn't know what was going on at all; stage three, when Dr. Horton starred with his ibuprofen hypothesis; and finally, stage four: the final, marvelous, brilliant inspiration about mastocytosis. The tone of the memo admittedly is a trifle boisterous. It sort of comes through that I am some kind of savant. At one point I say: ". . . primary systemic mastocytosis, a diagnosis which all of you missed---ho, ho, ho."

PETRIFIED

"Dr. Galen, here's Ms. Fogarty, back for her reports," says Sandra, beaming. Wonderful how she always beams (How can anybody beam at 10 a. m. on a heavy workday?)

Janet Fogarty bounces into the office in black corduroy slacks, white blouse, and a distinctly jaunty lateral hip movement. I tell her how normal her physical examination was and how beautiful the labwork is, and then I set myself to wondering what her main complaint was, the one that brought her here in the first place. I review the chart and note that she's had unaccountable pain in the thighs.

Examination showed no tenderness, no nodules, no thickening, no weakness, no varicositites, no nothing.

X-Ray, on the other hand, shows calcium deposits throughout the quadriceps, or thigh, muscles. The radiologist comments -- and I remember from pathology courses -- that this can be seen in a variety of conditions, including myositis ossificans, an unexplained disease in which muscles undergo degeneration, then calcium deposits there. It can also be seen in situations where trauma occurs. Trauma, of course, can come from repetitive injury.

"Ms. Fogarty," I say (it usually takes me about two meetings to call people by their first names if they are my age or less, and Ms. F. is about 18 years my junior -- she'll probably be Janet the next time) . . .

"Mrs. Fogarty" (I plug in the "r" in "Mrs." as soon as I've seen the "Married" instead of the "Widowed" or "Divorced" or "Single"-- I never liked this non-committal Ms. anyway) . . .

"Mrs. Fogarty, you have calcium in your thigh muscles, right about in the area where you hurt. Any chance you've injured your legs, or repeatedly injured them?"

"No, I can't think of any--"

"No automobile accident?"

"No."

"Or anything you do in your job?"

"Well, no, I just work as an insurance clerk at the Fidelity Company."

"Sit at a desk?"

"Mostly."

75

"What about at home? Any unusual hobbies?"

"No real hobbies. I don't have time, what with my after-hours work."

"After-hours work?"

"With the band."

"The *band?*"

"Tom's band. You know, mostly Latin music. Brazilian stuff -- *La Cucuracha,* that sort of thing."

"Janet" (notice how easily I've moved to Stage II) how often do you, uh, work with the band?"

"Oh, five nights a week."

"For how long at a time?"

"Maybe four hours, counting the gigs before and after intermission."

"And, Janet--exactly what do you do with this band?"

"I'm the tambourine player."

"And what do you do with the tambourines?" I'm beginning to sweat again. I really need a Gatorade dispenser around here.

"I shake them, and move around, and beat them against my legs, and--"

"*Beat* them against your legs."

"Yeah, you know--"

"Like maybe your upper legs?"

"Sure, my, you know, thighs. "

"Right where you hurt?"

"Well, yes, now that you mention it."

"Janet."

"Yes, sir?" (first time for that).

76

"You don't -- you don't actually have your tambourines with you, do you?"

"Well, no, not right here with me, but they're in the car."

"Any chance you could get them and show me exactly what you do? It might be important."

"Sure."

I punch the intercom key. "Sandra."

"Yes, sir."

"Mrs. Fogarty is going to her car and get her tambourines and come back and show me how she beats her thighs with them so I can determine if this is the cause of her myositis ossificans."

"I'm sorry, Dr. Galen, this intercom has been acting up and I really hope, I mean, I didn't *understand* that at all. What, please?"

"I said, Mrs. Fogarty will be coming back to see me in the office in a few minutes."

"Oh, yes, sir. Sure. I'll send her back when she returns."

ROUGH DRAFT

Irene hands me the typewritten memo about Diana Sorensen and the Great Inspiration.

"I decided to type that up in draft," she says, "in case you want to change anything."

"Draft? Change anything? What would I change?"

"Well, I don't know. I was looking at the first admission, you know, when she came in through the emergency room."

"Yes?"

"And right here it says, in your dictation, under 'Impression': it says, 'Primary systemic mastocytosis--'"

"I said that -- then? Wow, there I was, considering that possibility even in the middle of the night. What a whiz. Like I was telling Donna--"

"Dr. Galen, it says, 'primary systemic mastocytosis is an extremely unlikely possibility.'"

"Oh."

"And, Dr. Galen--"

"Yes?"

"There isn't any sign that you got a test for histamine then or looked back at the films or tested those freckles--until today."

I take the chart and the memo into my office and close the door again. I read the whole thing through. I decide to make one small alteration in the text. At the point where it says ". . . a diagnosis which all of you missed. . . ."

I change all of *you* to all of *us*. And I decide not to send a copy to Dr. Wahldenstrom.

After all, he's a very busy man.

And I make sure I didn't actually write down anything about being a savant. So I don't have to insert the word *idiot*.

TECHNIQUE

The intercom comes on. It has its own special static.

"Dr. Galen, this is Sandra. Mrs. Fogarty is back."

"OK, Sandra, send her in."

"Dr. Galen, (Sandra now in a stage whisper) you don't have anybody in the office with you, do you?"

"No, Sandra. Why?"

"Because Mrs. Fogarty is back here and says--

"Yes, Sandy?"

"Says she's going to demonstrate her technique for you."

"Yes?"

"And she has something with her, Dr. Galen."

"Yes, Sandra, what?" How I love being perverse.

"A pair of tambourines!"

"Send her right back, Sandra. And, Sandra."

"Yes, sir?"

"Close the door, please."

After this, the girls around the office will look at me a little different, maybe even treat me with a little more respect.

For about a week.

MIDLIFE CRISIS

Monty Lawrence's labile hypertension has luckily never been a real problem, and today his periodic blood pressure check is not bad -- 136/84. But by his slumped position and his downward gaze as he sits on the end of the examining table, I suspect he is feeling depressed.

I decide to use the "can opener." "Monty, is there something you want to tell me?"

The 45-year-old well-groomed computer executive looks at me, trying to decide if he can trust anyone with this. "OK, Doctor." Apparently he can trust it with me. "When I wake up in the morning I don't want to go to work. What's that song, turn left at Commerce Street or something, skip work, just head west? That's the way I feel. My marriage is not too rewarding. I'm nervous all the time. I don't sleep well any more. I must be having a mid-life crisis." By now he is sitting up a little straighter.

"Monty, it does sound that way. Now of course you know the mid-life thing was more common in the seventies and eighties and it's quite frankly not as much in style now. Nevertheless, I think you'll profit from my little instruction sheet which was developed during those critical years." I go to the wall desk, take out a printed page, and hand it to Monty. "Read this. I'll be back and we'll talk."

LIVING WITH THE MID-LIFE CRISIS
by John Galen, MD
(Male Version)

You are struggling with why this happened to you. Don't waste time with such analysis -- the causes for this syndrome are unclear. The point is -- the diagnosis and treatment are easy.
Sure, a whole lot of miscellaneous explanations have been proposed, including:
- male menopausal melancholy
- declining hormone levels
- topping out in your career
-grieving because you missed the sexual revolution
- fear of aging in a youth-oriented society

- your wife doesn't manifest adoration in every gesture

Don't get confused. Just pay attention to this plan. The key is: You must realize that there are major and minor criteria of the mid-life crisis. More important, since the syndrome is self-limited and goes away in about three years, the trick is to stay with the minor -- and avoid the major -- manifestations. The minor ones cause no lasting damage. The major ones are big trouble -- in fact, they are more dangerous than having the crisis in the first place.

Therefore -- you must inventory your lifestyle in multiple areas with this major/minor concept in mind:

SPORTS: Minor criteria -- taking up, for the first time at age 48, a vigorous sport like running, race-walking, skiing, or driving sports cars in rallies. These are transient things. Major manifestations include motorcycle racing, sky diving, and jumping off the cliffs at Acapulco. These can be permanent.

CLOTHING: Minor -- gold chains around the neck, pirate shirts open to the waist. Major -- wearing a Speedo bathing suit, estimated weight 2 grams, around anyone who knows your name. Minor -- wearing overalls to the doctor's office. Major -- wearing overalls to the doctor's office and you're the doctor.

ACCESSORIES: Minor -- wearing a toupee. Major -- wearing a toupee on your chest. Minor -- sunglasses indoors and out. Major -- calling them shades and wearing them outdoors at night. Minor -- going around the office with your wedding ring off. Major -- going around home *with your wedding ring off. Most Major -- going around the office and home with a ring in your* ear.

CAREER: Minor -- taking a sabbatical (like a year off in Britain to study Welch folkways). Major -- taking a sabbatical in Britain or anywhere without mentioning it to your boss. Minor -- quitting job such as sales manager and taking another, equal, job in an unrelated field, such as director of human resources.

81

Major -- quitting job such as sales manager and taking position of assistant dogcatcher in Aspen.

LOVELIFE: Minor -- telling 25-year-old woman you're in love with her. Major -- telling 25-year-old woman you're in love with her and it's true.

DRUGS: Minor-- getting bombed at Saturday night parties. Major -- getting bombed at power breakfasts. Minor -- puffing a little Mary Jane. Major -- agreeing to try crack because you thought it referred to the female anatomy.

MEDICAL: Minor -- thinking you need a psychiatrist. Major – actually going to one. Most major -- signing up for three times a week for five years. Minor -- face-lift. Major -- sex-change operation.

LANGUAGE: Minor -- using phrases such as "where you're coming from," "meaningful dialogue," and "getting into" something. Major -- using terms such as "getting into your dreams" and "rapping." Most major -- saying "like" before every fourth word and "you know" before every third. Example: "I really think I'm, you know, going to, like, split down to the, you know, store and, like, pick up some, you know, happy juice." You may not be able to recover after contracting this malady.

MISCELLANEOUS; Minor – subscribing to Playboy *for the first time at age fifty. Major -- subscribing to* Hustler. *Most Major -- letting Playboy, Hustler, or Sixty Minutes interview you.*

Careful attention to these distinctions between major and minor criteria can avert critical consequences of the crisis. Good luck.

"Did you read it, Monty?"

"Yes, Doctor, I read it, and it's amusing, but my problem is serious."

"Of course it is, Monty, because it's *your* problem. But did you get any message from that little sheet?"

"I guess something like: If I don't screw up real bad during this period of crisis everything will be eventually be all right."

"Very good, Monty. That's it exactly. This is the wrong time to make decisions about important things like your marriage and your job. You need to hang in there, get a Mazda Miata, put Brut on your face, stay away from drugs, minimize alcohol, eat sensibly, take exercise, and, most of all, wait."

"I'm sure you're probably right, John. And I am listening."

"Good, Monty. By the way, man," I said.

"Yes?"

"Where did you get those cool shades?"

THE PATIENT MAKES THE DIAGNOSIS

"In case you want to know, Karen Coberley is coming in at 2 p. m.," says Natalie.

"Good. What did you and Sandra and Karen do, have a full-scale conference call to work that big problem out?"

"Dr. Galen, it was no problem for at all for experienced health professionals like us."

"Don't know what I'd do without your expertise."

Natalie gives an abbreviated curtsey and returns to her office. Must be a strain to be on stage all the time.

REVISED TO HERE 8-28

And a strain it was, I recall, even to listen to Karen recount her history in that hospital room 25 years ago. Each element only served to confirm what I had already suspected -- and feared.

"I guess I was OK until about a month ago," she said. "Then I started noticing stiffness in some of my joints."

"Which ones, Karen?"

"Oh, my knees, wrists. Maybe just one at a time. Some mornings I'd wake up with stiffness in the little joints of my fingers -- isn't that weird, ever heard of that?"

"Yes, indeed," I said. *All too often.* "Then what happened, Karen?"

"Let's see, I had this sort of catching pain in the front of my chest."

"I see. Did it radiate anywhere? I mean, go from your chest to somewhere else?"

"Now that you mention it, it went up around my neck, like a collar."

"What was the effect of breathing?"

"It hurt to take a deep breath or lie down flat. Sometimes it hurt to swallow. It went away in about a week."

"I see. Then what?"

"Well I went to Dr. Mansfield. He said I had blood and albumin in my urine and a murmur. Made me come in here. Now you're going to spring me, right?"

"Patience, Karen. Any skin rash?"

"No -- unless you count that breaking-out I had last month after going to the beach."

"What part of your body broke out?"

"Oh, everywhere the sun hit -- you know, not under my bathing suit or anything."

"What else?"

"Let's see, I had some fever -- maybe 100-101. And Dr. Mansfield said I was anemic. I haven't felt all that great. But not too gross, either."

Not, probably, as gross as I felt at that moment. For, as usual, the history given by the patient was the key to the problem -- not scans, electrical monitors, radioactive blood studies. She had told me she had arthritis, pericarditis, fever, anemia, murmur, urinary abnormalities, sun-induced rash.

She had, in short, told me she had lupus.

SPECIAL DELIVERY

Natalie is the one to tell me. "It's here, Dr. Galen. The helicopter. You can look out the window and see the confusion on top of Building B."

I do, and it sure looks like confusion, but I know it isn't. The praying mantis of a helicopter is resting now atop the Celtic cross on the pad. The EMTs are carefully lifting the stretcher out. Two nurses are managing the IV tubing. Two orderlies are helping. Even Dr. Joe Middleton has made the scene, watching the picture evolve.

"Bye, Natalie. I guess I'll be late all day."

"What else is new?"

"Natalie, we've got enough news breaking here without your editorials."

"Just being a realist, Dr. Galen."

I move toward the emergency room, figuring to arrive about the same time they bring in Jimmy Treadway, now-famous tractor victim. We decided on the ER trauma room as the place to stabilize Jimmy before taking him to ICU.

We decided. Actually *Dr. Joe Middleton* decided. I called him because he's a great general surgeon, and general surgeons should always be the captain of the ship in a case of multiple trauma. Furthermore, like me, he is on call today for emergencies, and when he heard the news he figured his appointment book was filled up for the next 24 hours. Name: Jimmy Treadway.

Stabilize. That's a gentle euphemism for Find out what the problems are and do what you can before moving the patient to the next stop. The hope that Jimmy will become really stabilized anytime soon is a vain one.

As expected, despite the large size of the trauma room, I can't get in for the people. That's OK, because I'm not really needed at the moment – dialyzing him on the artificial kidney is way down the line.

I spy the charge nurse amid the forest of bodies. "Getting some labs and gases, Marcie?"

"Done, Dr. Galen – they're supposed to bring them in here to us in a few minutes."

"What do his vitals look like?"

"Not great. BP 80 systolic, pulse 140, cold and clammy, temp 101. Came in with a mask. But shallow respirations and O2 sat 70, so we intubated him without waiting for the gases. We're pumping in colloid and have 8 units of O negative blood on the way. Portable chest being done. Urine – about 30 cc of bloody stuff in the Foley bag. Since I guess he left the other hospital."

"What about his mental status?"

"Delirious. Moving everything. 'Course now he's sedated. . . . to get him on the respirator."

Joe Middleton steps out, folds his stethoscope and shakes his head. "Have to say he's got an acute abdomen. And an acute chest too. One of the cardio-thoracic people is coming over. We'll do a non-contrast CT if we can get him in the machine. Then we'll go to the OR if he's stable."

Joe looks around and then back at me. He lowers his voice a notch. "Or even if he's not."

"Acute abdomen" is a magic phrase when intoned by a general surgeon. It means that there is something bad going on inside the belly that can only be fixed by surgery. They don't usually say "surgery." They say "going to the OR" or "I've got to go in there." Jimmy may have a ruptured stomach or intestine or a lacerated liver or a broken spleen or several of the above and probably couldn't survive without some repair work. You should get his blood pressure up before operating but it may be that it will never come up without stopping the internal bleeding.

While waiting for the lab, I use my higher mathematical powers and start counting the people. One surgeon, one emergency physician, two respiratory therapists, three nurses, one radiology tech begging for help to position the patient. Three IVs in place. A respirator hooked to a tube going down Jimmy's throat. At the head of the bed, the portable X-Ray machine, a clunky contraption which has never been minimalized even in this reductionist era.

"Oops, Dr. Galen," says Marcie. "K+ is 7.5."

"What's the ph?"

"It's 7.16. pO2 78, pCO2 15."

The potassium level is life-threatening, acidosis is severe. "OK, Marcie, you know the drill – sodium bicarbonate, glucose, insulin, calcium drip."

"Sure – two amps of NaHCO3, 50 cc 50% glucose, 10 units regular insulin – all IV stat. Then 2 amps Calcium gluconate in 500 cc at 100 cc a minute. Recheck the K+ in about 30 minutes."

"Right. I could have stayed in the office."

"No, no. I like you holding my hand."

WHO ONLY STAND AND WAIT

Inside the ER is not the only place where Jimmy has drawn a crowd. There are 12 people in the waiting room, all "with" Jimmy Treadway. In a small town in this southern state, the store doesn't keep when somebody gets real sick. You go with them to the hospital in the city.

The first step is, Joe Middleton and I shake hands with everybody (they had all stood up when we came in, even the women). The second step is, we sit down. Sitting down means we don't have great news. But we can see this group already knows it.

"Jimmy is mighty sick," I start. "He's got serious chest and abdominal injury and his kidneys have shut down. He's still in shock despite everything that's been done so far. We've asked Dr. Middleton here to see him. Dr. Middleton is a surgeon and may have to operate. Joe, you want to tell them about it?"

Joe looks from face to face – Mildred the mother, sitting there stoic in her print dress with a Kleenex in her hand, Jack the father with his rawhide face and pressed overalls, two sisters with stretch pantsuits, and then the rest of the crowd – extended family, friends, and oh yes, the pastor. If you are from some bucolic paradise, the preacher always comes.

"His abdomen shows signs of major internal injury," Joe says, then thinks better of his prose. "I mean, he's hurt bad in his belly. We aren't sure what's broken, or bleeding, but we feel like we have to operate and find out, fix it if we can. First we're transfusing him, trying to get his blood pressure up and Dr. Galen is getting his blood chemistries in shape. But the operating room is the next step."

"What do you think his chances are, Doctor?" Jack, slouched, was solemn.

"Hard to tell at this point. I guess maybe 50-50 is about the best we can say right now." *We* – the eternal physician disclaimer. *I can't carry this burden alone. All of us doctors, nurses, therapists, lab techs -- we.*

"When do you think you'll be out of surgery, doctor?" one of the sisters asks.

"Several hours," says Joe. "Depends on what we have to do. Then he'll go to ICU – the Intensive Care Unit."

I don't have to wait for the next question. "You'll be able to see him then, when things have settled down. Maybe one or two of you will want to look in the emergency room right now before he goes to surgery." Mildred and Jack nod.

The preacher walks up. "Doctors, I know how busy you are. But do you have time for a short prayer?"

Joe and I look at each other. We stand and bow our heads.

We have time.

SPELLS . . . AND SMELLS

I walk into the next ER cubicle, I look at my watch, and then at Julie. "Only 35 minutes, Nurse. Only twice as long as advertised."

"Better than I expected, I can tell you," says the pert young woman. Her hair is freshly done, and it is bouncin' and beautiful like the ads say. Her smile has a glow. She likes her job, is good at it, and she has a fully representative supply of the modern female's cocky aspiration to ascendancy in the workplace. She, like so many others, announces it periodically with semi-serious aspersions upon her superiors. Many of these allusions obliquely suggest that the physician's expertise is less than, shall we say, perfect and sometimes inferior to their own (at times they're right). As, for example, in looking at an electrocardiogram just reviewed: "Don't those T waves bother you, doctor?" Or, after perusing a set of physician's orders: "Shouldn't this patient be monitored?" Or, in the confused patient: "Don't you want a drug screen?"

As one privileged to have made hospital rounds, while a boy, with my physician-father I can discern the difference a generation makes. At the old St. Christopher's the nuns and graduate nurses would, upon Dad's approach, rise stiffly as one. The rustle of the long. multi-pleated,

90

starched gowns recalled the sound of a rising covey of quail. Their attention was all on him, their work suspended. Knowing no other scenario, I presumed this reaction routine and was inadequately impressed at the time. Now you can walk into a nursing station unnoticed, the invisible man. Worse, you can get the feeling that everybody -- including the aides and the ward secretary -- are deaf: "How's Mrs. Jones?" Silence. "Has Mr. Wilson gone for his CAT scan yet?" You could be in the Black Forest. You might, as I once did, call the head nurse and decide to be jocular.

"Why won't anybody speak to me any more, Mrs. Mouton?"

Mrs. Mouton, I knew, had a sense of humor, but it seemed to be in the "off" position this morning. "Dr. Galen, you know we're busy. What can we do for you?"

"I was thinking maybe, you know, I could even start up a conversation or something."

"Love to, but you know we've only got eight hours to get all this work done."

"That's the trouble. Nurses work from shift to shift and a doctor's work is never done."

"True," she said, and a faint pursing of the lips signaled that her whimsical nature was now returning. "Doctors, I guess you'd say, are shiftless."

I just went back to the office.

But by far the most discouraging is a university medical center scene: "I'm Dr. Galen." (You've carefully left your stethoscope carelessly hanging around your neck.) "Is Mr. Tripp making any progress?"

"You're <u>who</u>?"

You explain you're the private physician, you know, family internist, and then you get that look which says, Oh, *LMD* (Local Medical Doctor) -- most dreaded of all designations. Maybe you should have pretended to be a visitor. On several occasions, when asked to see a patient in formal consultation at the university hospital, I have signed my name and appended the stigmatic "LMD" just to be smart. It never seems to get a laugh.

But what dominated my twelve-year-old senses in the halls of the old Catholic hospital was not by any means the superficial trappings of the power structure but the magical smell -- of alcohol, or ether, or whatever that strange pungency could be -- that conferred upon workers in this arena their aura of separateness. They were the select, imbued by vocational circumstance with exemption from ordinary travail, immunity to ordinary disease. They were endowed by virtue of intellect, hard work, and special commitment with capabilities which just ever so slightly transcended the mortal.

And their talisman was the smell. I would detect it in the clothes of my father when his wished-for homecoming finally came at seven or eight p. m. and he handed my brother and me our almost daily surprise -- a toy, a new toothbrush, an offering perhaps designed to expiate in some measure his faintly perceived guiltiness at long absences. But it was not the gift that provoked my expectation and generated the surge of youthful joy: it was *he*, Dad, the physician, the healer, the permanent missionary, the soft but strong man with the wonderful, powerful smell, the magician. He was the modern Pasteur, the reincarnation of the idolized scientist of old. Like, for example, Leeuwenhoek, inventor of the microscope.

Microscope! My father actually had one! Indeed, I would creep into his office whenever possible to look at that wonderful aging optical device, purchased second-hand by him as a genteely impoverished medical student. Greenish from oxidation, it was the symbol of special knowledge, knowledge not granted to many; of the vow of dedication, a vow incanted by only a few; of power -- say it, *power* -- draped like a cloak about the shoulders of the chosen. I kept that microscope, used it in medical school despite its technological antiquity, carried it jealously back and forth to histology lab like a star sapphire. I have it still, in a glass bell on the shelf.

"Well, Julie, among other things I've looked at Mrs. Andrus' X-rays, and there's no obvious break in her pacemaker wire. Have you been able to get the chemistries?"

"No the lab hasn't reported them yet."

"See, I've done my job and you haven't done yours."

Her smile signals that she is not intimidated. "They keep saying it'll be five minutes."

"How's the lady doing?"

"Fine. Oh, here comes the printout. Looks like everything's normal."

"Can I look at the numbers or am I permitted?"

"Dr. Galen, get off my case." She laughs and hands me the laser printed sheet.

She's right. Blood sugar normal. Electrolytes (blood mineral levels) within normal limits. Nothing there. "We'll have to admit her and watch her," I impart.

"But if everything's OK, and the pacer is OK, hasn't she just had a vasovagal reaction?" Julie is still the diagnostician.

"Maybe. But there are two things about gadgets like that pacer."

"What?"

"Number one, they're wonderful."

"Yes. And?"

"Number two, they're infernal. When you're in doubt about a machine, something's probably broke."

NAIL STRIPES

Back in the office, the book says I am to see Alicia for the first time, and I think back to the preliminary telephone conversation with her mother several days ago.

"Doctor, we don't want any stone left unturned," Mrs. Tannenbaum said. "We've got to get Alicia well, got to find out what it is that makes her keep changing weight so drastically. She's seen everybody without results, but we know you can do it, Doctor. They all say you're the man." Mrs. Tannenbaum, I thought, reminded me of my high-school track coach -- until he found out I was slow.

"How much weight fluctuation has she had, Mrs. Tannenbaum?"

"You wouldn't believe it. I'm embarrassed to say."

I wait.

"She has gotten down below 70 pounds and up to 200. And she's only 5-foot-four and 21 years old." Mrs. T. denied any significant abnormality of Alicia's dietary pattern, but I knew that didn't prove anything. In the peculiar area of eating disorders, surreptitious behavior is the rule.

Now Alicia herself comes into the office for an initial history. She is attractive, weighs 112 pounds, has an excellent figure, and is brightly outgoing. She has been admitted to the hospital on several occasions, twice for dehydration, malnutrition, and "electrolyte disturbances," and once for massive obesity. She says she is mystified at her massive weight fluctuations. She brings in assorted materials from previous doctor-visits, including blood chemistry determinations. We have a nice conversation, in which I try to make friends. I do not lean on her at this time for details of dietary history, for I know from experience that if I did so she would never even come back to complete the evaluation.

It is not necessary, anyway. Her blood chemistry studies from elsewhere not only are abnormal, they tell an undeniable story; they invade, in their insidious numeric way, her metabolic privacy. In every case, her serum potassium level is low. Sometimes she has alkalosis, sometimes acidosis: but always the low K+. A hard sequence to acquire without vomiting on the one hand, diarrhea on the other. My proposed preliminary scenario: overeating-->obesity-->guilt or self-consciousness-->induced vomiting and/or starvation periods and/or heavy laxative-taking. Name of syndrome? Polyphagia/bulemia/anorexia nervosa/laxative abuse. Cause? Essentially unknown (psychiatrists disagree). Treatment:

difficult. Prognosis? Not good; some even die. Here, as always, we'll give it our best shot. First, get the essential data. Second, try to get her confidence. Third, explain the situation in a non-accusative manner and try to work with a psychiatrist and the family over a long, long period of therapy. Sometimes even put down a nasogastric tube for feeding purposes.

Her physical examination is interesting in that it is completely normal except for two findings. The first is striae, or stretch-marks, over the lower abdomen, shoulders, and thighs. These are the tracks of rapid weight-gain, in which the under-layers of skin have been torn in the process of fat accumulation. It is also sometimes seen in weight-lifters whose muscles suddenly expand at a rate faster than the overlying cutaneous envelope can accommodate. Alicia's stretch-marks are old, new, and in-between. Up, down, up, down.

And the second finding is in Alicia's fingernails and toenails. They show -- all of them -- a series of white, slightly raised, transverse bands. I count them -- four stripes on each fingernail. Toenails, too. Pink, white, pink, white. These are Muercke's lines, named after the clever physician-observer who first recognized them and tied them to periods of protein depletion. But similar lines can occur in almost any condition of metabolic stress: heart attack, prolonged surgical episode, severe infection. Or, as here, profound weight loss. Since fingernails normally grow out from base to tip in about six months, Alicia's stripes tell me of four periods of starvation in the last 180 days or so. Poor child, she has no secrets from her physician.

Fingernails, indeed, can be a source of startling revelations. I think back to Harley Jackson, who came in from a neighboring state six years ago. He was a 33-year-old construction worker who was sent in to our hospital by his very good (and well-named) physician Dr. Earnest.

"Dr. Galen," he had said, "this boy is a mystery. Keeps getting very ill with abdominal pain, anemia, numbness in his feet. Comes in the hospital, we work him up. Looks like vasculitis or some other collagen disease. Two or three times we've treated him with steroids, each time he gets better, goes home, comes back within several months. We need help."

The house officers and student had examined Harley in some detail and presented all the available facts in the conference room. Then we went to the bedside, where I went over key elements of the history and physical examination.

"Harley, I said, we're going to have to do some more tests to pin this thing down. See you later."

Back in the conference room, I looked from intern to resident to medical student. I tried to keep the gloat out of my face.

"We're waiting for the labwork," said Jim, the junior resident.

"But we really already know the answer, don't we?" I enjoyed the blank stares for a moment. "The preliminary tests won't help, will they?" I relished the wonderful slackness of the jaws.

97

The senior resident spoke up. "I guess you're going to have to relieve our ignorance, Dr. Galen. We're striking out so far."

"His fingernails. Look at them later -- don't go back right now. Multiple transverse white bands. Episodes of abdominal pain. Neuropathy. Anemia. Weight loss."

The senior medical student, interestingly, was the first to brighten. "Mee's lines," he said. "Arsenic!"

The residents looked up, first at the student, then at me; seeing the approval in my eyes, they turned back to the student with grudging admiration.

After the tests, after the high arsenic level in the urine, in the fingernails themselves, in the slow-growing pubic-hair shavings, I was the one who had to tell Harley, the patient.

"You mean, Doc, I've been getting arsenic from somewhere?"

"On several occasions. Multiple doses over a period of time, then you'd come in the hospital and get better. Then you'd be discharged and get more arsenic, then get sick again."

"Damn. But where could I be getting the stuff?"

I didn't say anything.

"The little diner I eat lunch in every day?"

"Anybody else who eats there get sick?"

"No. Could I be getting the poison at home?"

Again I was silent.

He thought a long time. "Doc, I think I have some ideas. You know, my wife and I don't get along too well. We got divorced once and married again. She acts funny

98

sometimes.   And there's something else, now that I think about it."

"What?"

"I just took out a new insurance policy about 18 months ago. A good-sized one. About $100,000. And you know what?"

"What's that, Harley?"

"She's the sole beneficiary."

We treated Harley for his problem, which at the time included daily intravenous administration of British Anti-Lewisite, a drug with the property of forcing the poisonous metal out into the urine, and he went home. Later I heard from Dr. Earnest that he had pressed charges against his wife. A criminal trial ensued. She got off -- inadequate evidence, they said.

But, Dr. Earnest told me, Harley *did* get another divorce.

Indeed, fingernails can tell stories. Club-shaped nails from many conditions, including lung tumors (sometimes the clubbing goes away when the tumor is removed). Splinter hemorrhages in patients with endocarditis (heart valve infection). "Half-and-half" fingernails in patients with chronic kidney failure ("uremic poisoning"). This last has been the source of much professional satisfaction to me. For example, the patient is a white male, brought to the emergency room and deposited by agencies unknown. He is stuporous, his blood chemistries show kidney failure. No real history is available. The resident and intern wonder if he has been exposed to a toxin and hence has acute kidney shutdown.

You walk up, notice the brownish discoloration of the peripheral half of the fingernails and toenails. Seeing you have an audience, you may here, if you wish, fold your arms. It may be useful to shake your head and cluck softly. In any event, you will, by now, have their attention. It is usually preferable to be a trifle oblique.

"Nutrition not too bad for someone with chronic kidney failure of this duration," you might point out. Or, "Do the chronic dialysis people have any open slots right now?" Either comment will reliably cause pacing behavior on the part of the house officers.

"Well, sir, we thought we'd check things out and find out for sure if this is long-standing or acute first."

Here it is important to exhibit great patience. "That, of course, is a key step, but we've already taken that, haven't we?" You are having fun, but this scenario is not unmixed self-aggrandizement: after you have, at last, pointed out the critical physical finding, these youngsters will never forget the half-and-half phenomenon.

It is characteristic of teaching that the receiving end is 90 per cent of the process. You can convey the same ideas, say the same words, use the same inflections, keep the same gestures--and the results will vary 1:10 depending on the condition of the listening apparatus. The finest grass seed, broadcast widely over a parched plain, will expire without further biologic ceremony. Water the ground first, till it, make sure all the critical minerals and nitrogen are present, and the cheapest brand of fescue will germinate lasciviously.

So with learning. Give a monotonous lecture, crammed with facts, and count the glazed eyes. Read the didactic textbook aloud; and EEGs (brain wave tracings) applied to the medical students' heads would show a sleeping pattern.

No: first get yourself -- or any other student -- aching with that peculiar craving called curiosity. Feed it, tickle it, nudge it, titillate it. Bring it to a boil. Make the answer difficult to come by. Don't tell them. Yeats said education was less like filling a pail than lighting a fire. Send them to the library. Don't help them find it. Hope they struggle for a day or two. When the delicious answer surfaces, they will never forget. More important, they have sipped of the exotic liquid which will later become an obsession: they will search for the Pierian spring, seeking, seeking a niagara.

PBL

All of which reminds me of PBL. PBL stands for Problem-Based Learning. A few years back, I got to participate in a faculty committee to review the curriculum at Jones Medical School. I figured I was the token alumnus or token practicing physician among the full-time academics, many of whom were tenured. Anyway, they wanted to consider the possibility of reengineering the whole teaching system. I thought that was very innovative and admirable of the faculty until I heard the medical students come in and testify before the committee. They said they were bored to death, they had spent their lives listening to lectures, the lectures were terrible, and the attendance was down to 40% in some classes. Something needed to be done. So the wonderful inventiveness of the faculty was really student pressure. Among the solutions proposed -- and the one which was finally put into effect -- was the Problem Based Learning Concept. In this process, freshman and sophomore students are brought in, *de novo,* and given a case to solve. There were to be eight in a group, with one or two faculty mentors in the room. The facts of the case were fed stepwise over two or three sessions, and the students were to muck their way through the clinical enigma and the medical literature.

The faculty reaction was mixed, but three questions were raised. First, did the teachers have time to sit there while the students struggled through one case at a time? Second, won't the students have huge holes in their database with this hit-and-miss method? Will they pass their Boards? And third -- this one wasn't voiced -- could the faculty members really shut up while the students crept through the diagnostic and therapeutic pathways?

Anyway, it worked. In my sessions at least the students' eyes were wide and non-glazed. Their pupils were dilated. They couldn't wait to speak. It was Crossfire. When one adventurous student wandered out to sea, three others threw him a rope.

Says one: "This could be a stroke. We need to do an MRI."

"No, Neil," says another, "there aren't any local findings."

"Anyway," says still another, "you haven't done a good physical exam yet, why do you want an MRI?"

Students might escape their professors but never their peers.

The National Board scores actually improved, and the youngsters loved it. In one session, involving a complicated biochemical problem, one young man said, "This metabolic acidosis is so interesting I can't wait till we study intermediary metabolism."

"Really?" I asked.

"Yeah," he answered. "I may even go to class."

SOAP

Sometimes the Jones Medical School flatters me with an invitation to speak to the freshmen medical students as they start their very first year. It's a heavy responsibility because I'm up there with the Dean of the Medical School, the Dean of Education, and on occasion the President of the whole University. But the real pressure for me is not the dignitaries on the podium. It's knowing that I'm addressing an array of hothouse plants -- more than a hundred cautiously nurtured, meticulously selected, succulent flowers from the academic garden, all with dilated pupils and unlimited expectations. So, knowing the students are about to have -- the very next day -- their first live introduction to real patients down at the huge community hospital, I tell them about *Soap*.

Not the usual soap. And not the SOAP they will use as an mnemonic when they write up a patient -- that's Subjective, Objective, Assessment, and Plan; they will use, and curse, that system enough in due time. I mean the Soap they will use to let oil and water mix. Because most patients, unlike these students, do not have a background of leading their classes through 13 years of school; are not necessarily cultured, articulate, and driven. They are oil and the students are water -- the two layer out, immiscible, unless a detergent agent is added.

The agent -- the Soap -- I tell them, is *patience*. Not *-ts*, but *ce*. Then I recite a few of my own failures. The man who wanted his wife seen by "the head man at the clinic." Irritably, I said, "As far as we're concerned, that's me," only later realizing he meant a neurologist. The brand-new mother with a little protein in her urine whom I evaluated so thoroughly, only to learn that she later, in tears, described my visit as "a third degree."

This makes me think of Andy Doherty. It's hard to forget Andy. He came in one day, said he just wanted a physical, had no complaints. He was about 6'4", weighed 295, and his skin was very close to onyx. His hands were spade-like, calloused, and his body lacked the soft layer of adipose tissue just beneath the cutaneous envelope that nearly everybody has. Instead a carapace of muscle covered him – that had, on exam, the texture of anthracite. Andy operated a huge backhoe for a living; one wondered whether he or the machine had the stouter sinews. He exhibited a grinning, amiable way, perhaps because he had encountered few arguments in his time.

After the checkup, I told him everything looked good, and we'd just do a few tests. But I could see he had something else to say. Often the end of the exam tells you what brought the patient in. His wife sent him? His boss? The guy next door dropped dead? A fear of cancer?

"Thank you, Doctor." He looked at the floor and shook his head, smiled, and then shook his head again.

I decided it was Soap time. "Got something else on your mind, Mr. Doherty?"

"Doctor, everybody just calls me Andy. Well, yessir, I guess so. If I'm in pretty good shape, I was just wonderin.'"

"Wondering what, Andy?"

"Do you think I'm a candidate?"

"A candidate, Andy? For what?"

"For some of that there Vigoro."

PROGRESS NOTE

I'm standing in the office hallway thinking deep thoughts about disease and life, like whether I might make the symphony tonight, when Natalie hands me the cell phone.

"Marcie, Dr. Galen. Jimmy Treadway. K 6.5 now. T waves still peaked on EKG, but the P waves look more normal."

"Good. Well, not good, but better. Why don't you repeat the bicarb and keep up the calcium drip."

"I'll tell them — you know, he's already in the OR. They've just started."

"Do you know what his vitals are now?"

"They say systolic BP is 90. Dr. Jackson Martin, the thoracic guy, put in a chest tube before he left the ER."

"Get much fluid out?"

"Two liters of bloody stuff and bubbles. I guess he had a pneumo too."

Translation: Blood pressure slightly better/ they're getting ready to make an incision in his belly/ a lot of fluid and blood was in his chest cavity/ his lung has a hole in it/ air is loose inside the chest/ the lung is partially collapsed /the chest tube is dealing with it.

"And now, Marcie, I guess you're going to give me the good news?"

"Sure. Nice day out there."

"Great."

"And then too, Dr. Galen . . ."

"Yes?"

"Jimmy's still alive."

HIPAA

"I don't get this at all, John," says U. S. Senator Pete Callahan. He is seated in one of the two orange leather chairs which have added the only dash of color to my office for about 30 years. He is here for a brief follow-up check on his blood pressure and cholesterol following a recent hospital admission for a gallbladder removal. And he is perturbed about something.

"I mean, the hospital was fine and the surgery went great. Can't believe they can just stick that little tube in through a half-inch incision, pull the whole gallbladder right out, send you home the next morning. But they told everybody in the whole world about my medical problems. Without my permission. The insurance company. The

106

federal government. They even reported my tests to a CDC database."

He leafed through several sheets of paper. "Everybody in the world, that is, but my wife. She couldn't find out anything. She heard -- from my office -- I had gone in unexpectedly, called up the hospital, was told they couldn't release any information. She just asked, 'Is Senator Callahan even in the hospital?' Got back, 'Can't tell you that. Government regulations.' So on. Had to call your office, track you down, just to locate my body."

"I remember, Pete. And of course I talked to Adele, brought her up to date."

"Well, I appreciate that."

"You mean, particularly since I broke the law and risked prosecution? You're a lawyer, you know what that means"

"John, what the hell are you talking about.?"

"I'm talking about the HIPAA provisions."

"Which are?"

"That the hospital or doctor cannot release a single fact to a friend or relative without the patient's written release. Not to the spouse, not to the son. Our office computers have funny lined screens so that passersby can't read them. Of course the personnel using the computers can hardly read them either. Federal law. I'll show you one, if you like."

"Never mind, John, never mind. But then the hospital turns around and sends out my whole medical record to, let's see . . . " He shuffled some paper. " . . . Aetna, the Federal Congressional Insurance Program, the Treasury Department,

God knows what else. I guess my opponent in the upcoming election could get hold of it."

"Maybe so. HIPAA in action."

"My opponent, but not my wife? OK, then, what the hell is HIPAA?"

"The Health Insurance Portability and Accountability Act. Sounds good, eh?"

"When in God's name was that passed?"

"In 1997."

"And it's just now getting enforced, 6 years later?"

"Your government in action."

"But I never signed any releases to send stuff to all those agencies."

"Don't have to. Read the regs. The hospital is obligated to do it on request. You can't even stop them. You're practically on the internet."

"That's crazy. What else is in those regs?"

"Lots. Doctors have to put down all the right words to justify a Medicare exam or they may get fined, accused of fraud. Any pattern of errors can be extrapolated over the entire practice. I know of a group of kidney doctors who had an FBI team come in, offer to fine them 10 million dollars. They appealed it, one of the docs spent three years in court. Got the fine down to 1.2 million plus community service. You read the bill, it sounds like they're talking about drug lords instead of doctors."

"My God, John, this is America. That sounds like jack-booted, brown-shirted Wehrmacht tactics."

"The similarity is striking."

"I'm going to go back and raise some hell about that in Washington."

"Good."

"How could that have ever passed?"

"My question exactly."

"I'll find out who-all voted for it."

"Let me help you."

"Who, then?"

"Everybody."

"What do you mean?"

"Isn't this your second term?"

"Yes."

"So you were in the Senate in 1997?"

"Yes."

"The vote in the Senate was 100-1."

"Really?"

"Everybody voted for it, Pete." I shifted in my chair. "Including you."

THE THRILL IS GONE

"Karen Coberley's in Room 4," says Donna. "Fistula doesn't look so good. Probably needs declotting."

"Thanks a lot, Doctor Donna," I reply. "You wanna' call the vascular surgeon now? Or should I stick my head in the room just for the record?"

"Whatever you say. But there's no thrill, no bruit." Donna's head is tilted to one side, her eyes are directed heavenward, her arms are outstretched, palms upward. Her patented flush, involving arms and neck as well as face, returns. Donna is so abused, her body English says, so longsuffering. After all, the absence of the little whirring noise and the little buzz over Karen's artificially created arterial-venous connection in her arm can only mean one thing -- it's stopped up. A medical technologist can tell that, can't she? It can't be used for the regular three-times-a-week dialysis unless the clot is removed. And it needs to be removed right away, doesn't it?

Fact is, I already know Donna is right. And she knows she's right. And she knows I know she's right. Furthermore, I see the surreptitious wink she throws at Natalie as she walks back to the lab.

On the way to Room 4, I recall Karen's reaction, at age 15, in the University Hospital, to the news that we had to change her diagnostic label.

"I think you have just one problem," I said, trying to dress it up a little for teen-age consumption. "Not rheumatic fever plus glomerulonephritis, but another single disorder. We'll need more tests before we can be sure."

"Heck," she said, "that sounds better. Doesn't it?"

"We'll see," I answered, using the doctor's all-purpose dodge. And doing anything I could to avoid, or at least to defer, the use of the word *lupus*. For as soon as that voodoo chant is uttered, nothing is ever the same again. Family members scatter: to the dictionary, to the popular medical book, to the internet, to the family physician, to a friend whose cousin is supposed to have the disease. Only the worst news comes back: Lupus kills. It ruins your blood. It destroys your kidneys. You bleed to death. It makes young

110

women look like a wolf. I have had patients, newly aware of their diagnosis, discuss it with a best friend and be told: "Lupus! Good God! You're going to die!"

No, friend, you don't use that word until you're sure. And as soon as you do, you must be ready then and there to do a detailed education job. You must prepare the patients for the onslaught of street knowledge which will surely besiege them. They must know more than anyone else. They must be comforted by the power which is only bestowed by abolition of the unknown. They will march into their family room, their classes, their workplace, their cocktail party armed against casual and careless comment with the only weapon which is effective: authentic learning.

Lupus -- technically disseminated lupus erythematosus -- is a disease of autoimmunity in which the body behaves as though it is attacking itself. Antibodies form against various normal tissue constituents, such as nucleoproteins. Thus the skin may break out -- the butterfly rash over the bridge of the nose is classic. The joints may develop inflammation. Blood components may be affected -- the white count goes down, with resultant decreased resistance to infection; red blood cells may be prematurely disrupted or inadequately produced, leading to anemia; the platelet count may drop, producing a bleeding tendency. The pleural or pericardial surfaces may become irritated, causing pleurisy or pericarditis with pain and fluid accumulation. There may be unexplained fever. The central nervous system may be affected: strokes, seizures, psychosis may ensue.

111

Most of all, especially in young patients, the kidneys may be damaged. Like innocent bystanders, the tiny glomerular capillary networks unknowingly filter the disastrous load of circulating antigen-antibody complexes; their microscopic waste disposal mechanism, called the mesangial system, is overloaded. The capillaries themselves undergo changes, eventually are obliterated. Protein leaks into the urine. Swelling occurs all over the body. Kidney function declines. Uremic poisoning appears. The patient these days becomes a candidate for the artificial kidney or transplantation. But in those days, when Karen and I were talking in the room of the old Jones University Hospital, there was no chronic dialysis, no transplantation available.

For some strange reason, lupus affects women 20 times more frequently than men, and it particularly selects young women. Even more bizarre is the predilection of the disease for red-headed people. Sunlight usually aggravates the disease. So a young Titian-haired woman with a rash across the nose after exposure to the sun, joint pains, and albumin in the urine is a prime suspect.

And for some other strange reason, lupus, like other collagen diseases, waxes and wanes. Full-blown cases one year may elude diagnosis the next. The patient may have arthritis, then be well for a decade; anemia, then feel fine for years; pleurisy, then remit for months. Or all the manifestations may fulminate at once.

Fortunately, despite popular knowledge, and despite the lack of a cure, there is effective treatment. Cortisone derivatives and so-called immunosuppressive drugs can be

112

marvelously effective. Under good management, eighty per cent of lupus patients do well eighty percent of the time. They may even have a normal life expectancy, a high quality of life.

Then as now, the diagnosis of lupus depends on putting together all the clinical and laboratory manifestations to see if a definitive pattern emerges. Then as now, there was no single conclusive test, but these days we have a battery of serologic studies which greatly assist in diagnosis -- the antinuclear antibody test, the anti-DNA antibody assay, and others.

In Karen's case, at that time, the only blood test available which was reasonably specific was the LE cell prep. This peculiar test, discovered like so many others by accident, had to do with the tendency of normal white blood cells to develop strange patterns on incubation with serum from lupus patients. In Karen's case it was negative, but I knew this proved nothing; the LE cell phenomenon could come and go and was only valuable when positive.

So we were stuck: where to go from here? The next step, I knew, was probably a renal biopsy, in which a needle is inserted through the back into kidney tissue and a one-inch core about the size of a ball-point refill is obtained for microscopic analysis. Before considering this step, however, the patient's mother, the referring physician – and I -- decided to seek consultation at a big Eastern medical center. In fact, I was relieved to have a further opinion.

The problems with patients journeying to medical meccas, however, I knew, were two: (1) there is no magic at the other end, only good, orthodox methods; and (2) the patient can get lost in the system and never see the critical consultant. To avert these concerns, I referred Karen specifically to Dr. Paul Turnbull at the William Henry Research Center. He, I knew, was a gifted diagnostician, a thorough clinician, and, not inconsequentially, a fine fellow. He would get the answer or get someone who could.

He was also a world-class diplomat. He called me two days after Karen arrived.

"Doctor Galen, thanks for sending this lovely young woman. I agree with your diagnosis. She had the consideration to convert her LE Cell prep to positive on the train." Not, *Don't you guys know how to do these tests?* I'd like to nominate him for the UN job.

"Karen, you must be sick of seeing me," I now offer as I close the door of Room 4 behind me.

Her reply is characteristic -- she extends both her arms for a hug. "Dr. Galen, I can't stand being sick but I'll never get tired of seeing you." Some people seem to know just what to say.

I pick up her left hand and hold it out to the side. On the inside of her upper arm there is an irregular rope-like-like protrusion under the skin, as if an uncoiled snake has been implanted there. The fistula. The vascular access. The connection between the artery and vein which is the lifeline for the hemodialysis patient like Karen. It allows her to have needles implanted three times a week so that her blood can be cleansed, so that she can be reasonably well instead of chronically poisoned.

But today the snake, normally pulsatile and soft, normally possessed of a palpable buzz, or thrill, is hard and still. The stethoscope, which should transmit a rhythmic conch-shell roar, today delivers only an ominous silence.

OK, so Donna was right.

"It's stopped up, Karen. We'll have to get Dr. Rhine to work on this."

"That's what I figured. And I believe Donna thought so, too."

Some people just don't seem to know the right thing to say.

LAST DITCH

"How are you doing, Jimmy?"

"Great, Dr. Galen, just great. My business is going fine. Wife and baby are doing well. 'Course you know the baby is adopted."

"Sure. Let's see, Jimmy. We've been following you since . . . "

"Twenty-eight years ago. That's when I first saw you at Jones University Medical Center."

Incredible. Twenty-eight years ago Jimmy York was referred in for a "last-ditch" workup. Last-ditch, that is, before being consigned to a mental institution.

"John, I wish you'd look at this boy once before the family commits him," Dr. Waldo Cronk had said over the phone from Redville, S. C. "He's been out shooting guns at night, disappearing for days. He's impossible to control. Gets confused. Of course he's had the history of liver trouble, a congenital form of cirrhosis. Had a splenectomy and splenorenal shunt for varices. All that seems stable, but the behavior situation is out of hand. Question is, of course, whether it's purely psychiatric or whether there's an organic component."

"Maybe he has a little bit of hepatic encephalopathy or whatever," I said. "Send him down. We'll admit him and see what we can find out."

Funny how a doctor will say *we* when only referring to himself. Even a fellow in a one-man office will say, "We'll see what this medication does." (Here maybe *we* means the patient and the doctor together.) But also "We'll get you back in a month and see how things are going," or "When did we see you last?" (the receptionist, the secretary and I?), or "When did we see you in the emergency room?" Some wags (non-MDs, of course) have suggested it's the royal *we*, since doctors are supposed to be so haughty. Or maybe the editorial *we*, since we are so opinionated. I've always thought it was a syntactical mechanism by means of which to diffuse the terribly singular responsibility of being a physician into a more tolerable plurality. "Let's get you on blood thinners, Mr. Smith, and see if we can't prevent any more trouble" (*translation: I have accepted for you the weighty risks of anticoagulant therapy, including bleeding into shock from the intestinal tract or into trauma sites in the event of an accident, in the hope of preventing any more clots from leaving your fibrillating heart and ending up in your*

116

brain. I have explained this to you, of course, and have asked you what you want to do, but we both know it is I who make this decision. I am the one who carries this aching compromise home, to contemplate before the TV, to try to put aside while I study, to force back into the subconscious at four a. m. when the bad spirits come and nudge my shoulder). We then, is not royal nor editorial but euphemistic. It is a softening device, a psychic escape route. It is the back door.

But Jimmy York is a lesson in keeping the front door of your mind open. It was near the end of the day when I wandered up to 5-East at the University Medical Center, where Jimmy had been admitted to a semi-private room, now more than a score of years ago. The intern had seen him and had finished his notes, but it was the medical student, Roland Hampton, who accosted me as soon as I reached the floor.

"Dr. Galen, Dr. Galen, he's got Wilson's disease!"

"Sure, Roland. Come on into the conference room and let's sit down and you first tell me what Wilson's disease is." I was probably fairly patronizing at this point, since we were talking about an incredibly rare disorder of copper metabolism. It causes copper deposits in many organs, but it is the liver, brain and kidneys which bear the brunt of the disturbance. The metal also collects at the periphery of the colored halo around the pupil, a finding originally described by two physicians named Kayser and Fleischer.

Roland reviewed the basic characteristics of the disease fairly competently, then I asked him to tell me just which ones Jimmy York had.

"Well, he has the liver disease."

117

"Yes," I said. "We can get the original slides and review them. What else?"

"And he has the mental problems."

"Yes. Go on."

"And the tremor."

"I see."

"And, Dr. Galen, and--"

"Yes?"

"He has the Kayser-Fleischer ring!"

Later I felt impelled to call the chief of medicine and tell him about Roland's triumph -- after the copper was demonstrated in the liver on special stains, after the opthalmologist confirmed the nature of the ring on slit-lamp examination, and after fancy blood tests showed that Jimmy indeed had the typical defect of Wilson's disease -- absence of ceruloplasmin, the copper-binding protein. Jimmy was treated with penicillamine, a drug which drags the copper out of the body into the urine, a low copper diet, and potassium sulfide, which helps prevent dietary copper from being absorbed in the first place. He required a month in a psychiatric ward, but here he was now, still on his medicine, no problems with the liver and his brain working fine.

Now I look at his eyes with the office oph-thalmoscope. "The ring is still gone, Jimmy. We'll check the other tests and give you a report by telephone."

"Fine," says Jimmy. "Dr. Galen, have you ever heard from Roland Hampton, the medical student who first diagnosed me?"

118

"Yes, I have. Matter of fact I talked to him the other day about another patient."

"Oh, good. How's he doing?"

"Fine."

"What line of work did he finally go into?"

"You won't believe it."

"Tell me."

"Psychiatry. Maybe he's looking for more cases of Wilson's disease."

Jimmy nods, walks out to the reception room, scoops up his little boy, takes his wife by the hand, and goes shopping.

HABEAS CORPUS

Time for one phone call before the next patient.

"How are you, Miss Andrews?" (probably young enough to call "Jessica.")

"Fine, Dr. Galen. I was just wondering, how did my physical turn out?"

I remember that in criminal law, they can't keep anyone in prison without a good reason. The doctrine of *habeas corpus* (literally translated "have the body") protects the citizen from such treatment: his lawyer can demand that the prisoner be brought to court and that the state explain what's happening. Lots of people have been freed on the basis of this principle.

Jessica makes me realize there's a *habeas corpus* doctrine in medicine, too. She is a young teacher, actually in the health field. She had her blood and urine checked at a

119

nearby facility, got a chest x-ray, sent the reports to me, and now she wants to know all the answers.

I decide to be firm. "You haven't *had* a physical yet."

"But I sent you all my reports," she responded. "What's my cholesterol and blood sugar?"

"I will read you those figures, but I can't tell you if you have a gallbladder problem, or lumbar strain, or heart trouble, or early emphysema, or cancer of the cervix, or an enlarged liver. In short, I can't tell you if you're healthy or not without -- *habeas corpus*."

"Without what?"

"Without actually seeing you."

"But I thought that chemical profile would give all the key data. Maybe I'll come by and let you examine me sometime. How long will that take, about ten minutes?"

"Longer than that," I say. "You see, the main thing is not even the physical examination itself but the history."

"You mean, just talking to me?"

"Right. What you tell the doctor and how you tell it and how you answer his specific questions is the most important thing in your health picture. That was true in 1900 and it's true now. We have a lot of gadgets now we didn't have then, but the principle is the same. Let me tell you a story, if you have time, Jennifer.

Apparently she does. "A 31-year-old woman named Alice came in to see me last week after several years' absence. For four months she had been having back pain. She had been in to several drop-in clinics, had seen several doctors in her HMO. She'd seen a urologist and an orthopedist. She'd had back x-rays, kidney x-rays, even an MRI, a good many blood tests, taken a variety of anti-inflammatory medications. But she was no better, she was worse. She reminded me of you, Jessica: she said she guessed she hadn't had the right tests yet.

"I told that lady, Alice, that the main tests she needed were a history and physical examination. So she came in. "'What,' I asked, 'makes this pain better and what makes it worse? Does movement aggravate it? Does rest relieve it? Have you had any burning on urination?'"

"'Well,' she said. I haven't had any burning. Moving doesn't affect it. This is crazy, Dr. Galen, but the thing that makes it worse is getting hungry and the thing that makes it go away is eating something.'

"I had her twist and bend and stoop and stretch. None of these activities bothered her at all and she showed no limitation whatever. Clearly she didn't have a muscular or skeletal problem. What Alice did have, Jessica, was now pretty obvious."

"What, Doctor?"

"She had a peptic ulcer, probably on the rear part of her duodenum causing reference of pain to the back. But only talking to her and examining her brought it out."

"How's she doing now?"

"Fine. Upper GI series confirmed it. She responded immediately to treatment with diet, antacids, and a drug called cimetidine."

"Isn't that the medicine that stops acid formation in the stomach?"

121

"Yes."

"Maybe I ought to take that. Sometimes I wonder if I have an ulcer."

"Now you know how to find out."

"How? Get a, what, GI series?"

"Maybe. But mainly we need *habeas corpus*."

"What?"

"See your doctor. Jessica, what I mean is --"

"Yes, Dr. Galen?"

"Bring the body."

FOGGY BREAKDOWN

"Mrs. Patton is here, Dr. Galen. She brought the drug bottle," Sandra says. Sandra is chewing gum and trying to disguise it: she has it way over to the side of her mouth where she thinks it won't interfere with her speech. But you can hear the *Mrs. Baddon* and the *dug bodda.*

"Good. Show her in."

Mrs. Patton looks a little pallid. She walks in and dumps the contents of a small brown paper bag on my desk. "I think it's just what you suspected, Doctor."

Harold Patton is an old patient of mine. I was sort of proud of myself for finding the basis for his kidney disease more than sixteen years ago -- high blood calcium ("hypercalcemia")--which after much investigation proved to be due to taking in too much milk and alkali for the esophageal irritation deriving from his hiatal hernia. Since then his kidney disease had progressed slowly, and I knew -- and told him -- that at some point he would have to resort to dialysis or transplant. Two days ago he came in for a routine check: Blood urea nitriogen (BUN) and creatinine were rising, but nothing unexpected. I placed him on a vitamin and a phosphate binder known as Dialume. Then, yesterday at six a. m. -- forty-eight hours later -- I received a call from Mrs. Patton.

"He's just not himself, Doctor. He can't stand alone. Hot and sweaty. Talking out of his head. I don't know what to do."

I told her to bring him in, of course, and things were pretty much as advertised. For the first time since I had known him he was inattentive, distracted. His mental processes were foggy. I told Sandra at the time that he was acting like someone with hypoglycemia, as in an insulin reaction, but that he had no possible reason for such a condition. I assumed it was early uremic syndrome (sometimes called "uremic poisoning"). I ordered stat labwork and admitted him to the hospital. In about 40 minutes the lab called with the results: high BUN, high creatinine, high uric acid -- all compatible with his chronic kidney disease -- but also a blood sugar value of 31, which was very low, and not compatible with anything we knew of. In any event the nurses and I rushed to Harold's bedside, started an intravenous line, and began giving him concentrated glucose solutions. He perked up in minutes and said he felt fine, if a little weak.

"It couldn't be the medicine, could it, Doctor?" Mrs. Patton asked.

I assured her, probably rather pontifically, that, no, it really couldn't: one was just a multivitamin pill and the other was Dialume, a phosphate binding agent which did its work without even being absorbed from the gastrointestinal tract.

"That's the little blue pill, isn't it?" she said.

"Little blue pill? No, no, not a blue pill. It's a large, white one. Joan, when are you going home?"

"Why, tonight, Doctor."

"And when are you coming back?"

"In the morning. Why?"

"Would you bring those medications with you?"

And here they are now, in colorful array against the black desk-top blotter: the Iberet-Folic 500, a multi-purpose vitamin that had the advantage, unlike many such preparations, of containing the B-vitamin known as folic acid. And the blue pill -- not Dialume at all, but Diabinese. *Diabinese* -- an anti-diabetic medication, one designed to lower a high blood sugar to normal. But also one which, given to the wrong patient, or given in excess, can drop a normal glucose value to levels which will produce lethargy, coma, or even death.

Harold Patton, already sick enough from chronic renal failure, had been poisoned.

I pick up the bottle, labeled Haddonville Pharmacy, and move to get Harold's chart. I move with a ball of nausea growing in my midsection, threatening to rise at any moment into the throat and send me to the nearest receptacle.

Sandra hands me the chart. I open it to the last visit. The last line of the progress note reads:

124

"Disposition: Iberet Folic-500 I qd
Dialume, 500 mgm tid with meals"

Clear enough. But is it? The papers have been full of reports lately about physicians' illegible handwriting being responsible for wrong medications. It will be a matter of opinion, and it will probably be impossible to get the original prescription from the pharmacist.

Then comes Sandra, ah, Sandra: "I made a xerox copy of the prescriptions, Dr. Galen, like I always do."

Xerox! Sandra! Migraine! How wonderful!

Or is it? Is it wonderful? Is it, maybe, *horrible?* Like sweating out a blackjack hand for your life savings at a Las Vegas table I slowly uncover the sheet with the actual handwritten scripts. There's not much doubt.

Dialume is written, or scrawled, very legibly.

Diabinese? Hardly. My relief is palpable. I call in the entire office staff. They confirm: yes, my handwriting is not suitable for a calligraphic model, as they keep reminding me; but yes, this is actually better than usual; no, there is no possibility of confusing the inscription for Diabinese. I have Debra take it to three pharmacists and ask them to identify it. They agree.

Then I call the drug store which filled the drug request.

"I don't usually work here, just filling in. Let me get the original prescription." A pause. "Oh, yes, I can easily see how she would have confused this for Diabinese. That's how *I* might have filled it."

"You *would*?"

"Yes. I don't even know what Dialume is. She wouldn't either. Diabinese is what it looks like."

"And at that dose? *Three to six* times the usual starting dose?"

"Well, that's the way it's written."

"Have the pharmacist who filled this call me, please."

That was the trouble with Watergate. Not the sorry motives. Not the sloppy execution. Not the defamation of the U. S. political character which it implied. The American public, charitable to a fault, would have forgiven it all. "We've made a silly, terrible mistake," the president could have said, and he would probably have been covered with a mantle of warm grace. What they couldn't stand, of course, was the cover-up. Or the attempt at it.

And neither can I, now. My self-righteous indignation flames, kindled doubtless by the delicate tinder of my own close call, my own almost-self-pity, my own near-culpability. I am guilty myself, like the Watergate inquisitors, of that form of disdain which can only stem from an opportunity to be holier-than-you-know-who: anybody available.

But before I can get fully righteous or even indignant Sandra walks to the door and says, with just a trace of Thespianism:

"The pharmacist, Dr. Galen. The pharmacist at the Haddonville Drug Store, who filled Mr. Patton's prescription, is now on the phone for you." Stage directions call here for head and eyes to avert left as she exits. She complies.

"Doc-doc-tor Galen *(sniff),*" says the young feminine voice, "is-is-is-Mr. Patton-is he is he all right? *(sob, sob*") Oh, I've made a terrible *(sob)* mistake. Do you think he will -- will he recover? *(sniff)*?"

Gone is the crusading Watergate mentality. Auto-holiness, that deep, comforting sense of newly-acquired, synthetic piety, evaporates like the print on an electronic screen. Gone is the arrogance, a rush of human lacrimal secretion dissolving it as cleanly as handwriting on a glistening Atlantic beach at flood tide.

"He's fine as far as the medicine is concerned. Don't you worry, my dear, he's got a lot of problems, but from here on nothing you've caused. "

"Can-can I call him?"

"Sure, honey. Call 350-1335. He or his wife will probably answer."

ADMINISTRATIVE DETAILS

Natalie appears magically in the doorway. "Dr. Galen, can you talk to Dr. Rhine, now? He's on 3699."

I punch the blinking button and pick up the phone.

"Dan? What's up?"

A female voice comes on. "Hold for Dr. Rhine, please."

This whole process is getting worse all the time. You're Dr. A. You tell your secretary to get Dr. B. She gets Dr. B's secretary. Dr. B's secretary tells her she'll get him, but first get Dr. A on the line. Your secretary tells Dr. B's secretary she will, but get Dr. B first. Both secretaries stay on the line while new calls pour in and stay on hold. Dr. B arrives at the telephone first and waits for you (remember -- you're Dr. A). He gets tired of waiting and asks his secretary to hold. You come on and Dr. B has to be summoned. Finally you're both on the phone and you're both irritated. Both secretaries are irritated. The patients waiting for someone to answer are irritated.

"About Karen Coberley," says Dan Rhine.

"Right. Thanks for seeing her right away."

"No problem. We'll have to declot this thing."

"Yeah, I -- er, we -- figured."

"Thought we'd bring her in, do a regional block, maybe keep her overnight, make sure it stays open."

"Sounds good. We'll find her room number on the computer. She going straight to the OR or to outpatient surgery?"

"Probably the OR. Soon as they can work her in."

"We thank you and she thanks you."

Now Donna materializes. "What did Dr. Rhine say about Karen?"

I consider this question for a moment.

"Nothing much."

"Nothing much? Are you kidding me?"

"What do you think?"

128

"I think you're kidding me."

"Yeah. Otherwise I'd have to admit you were right."

"Well, we certainly wouldn't want to do that." She cranks up her flush again and turns to leave, but this time she's smiling broadly.

Before Karen needed this fistula in the first place, I recall, a whole lot of water had passed under her particular bridge. After her return from the William Henry Center, we started her on prednisone, 20 mgm. a day, and she blossomed. Her fever went away, her joint aches disappeared, her urine cleared, her anemia corrected, and even her LE cells disappeared. We tapered her down to 7.5 mgm. a day, then eventually put her on 10 mgm. every other day, a program designed to minimize side effects. Nowadays we'd probably do a renal biopsy anyway, classify the pattern of kidney trouble, decide if she needed another agent like cyclophosphamide or azothiaprine. But she straightened out on our minimal treatment. She continued her usual pattern in school, which included making straight A's, and decided to enter college, take pre-law, eventually go to law school, become a courtroom attorney. She thought she'd like litigation.

"I like to explain things to people," she had told me. "If you explain it just right, amazing how they'll agree with you."

Big plans. But there was a big problem: the local Jones University scholastic advisor said she'd never be accepted in its highly-rated law school, not with lupus. Her "physical outlook was too poor." I wrote letters to the President of the University, the Dean of the law school, the Dean of the College of Arts and Sciences. No soap.

Paul Turnbull even leaned on the people at William Henry University, where he was on the medical faculty. Not reasonable, they said, to take Karen what with all the other well-qualified candidates who were all healthy. No go.

Karen cried a little, and then got in State University, taking pre-law. I don't know if she minimized the health portion of her application. Knowingly, she never asked me to fill it out -- maybe she thought I had too much information. Anyway, she managed a 4.0 average through four years and got in the School of Law at State. The course was only two years then and she graduated at age 23 -- first in her class.

Then, after a struggle with questions of health certificates and non-insurability, she wangled a neophyte job with Hughes, Wyndham, and Smith, one of the top three law firms in the city.

The rest, Karen made sure, was history. I learned from friends in the legal business that her case preparation from the beginning was superb, her courtroom demeanor near-magic: judges and juries alike fell under her sway within minutes. Her handling of tort cases became a small regional miracle. There were 125 first-rate lawyers at Hughes, Wyndham, but clients stood in line down there waiting for Karen.

At 26 she was simultaneously the first woman, and the youngest person, to become president of the state bar association.

I thought all this was interesting news, so I wrote a letter outlining the developments, complete with newspaper clippings, to Dr. Paul Turnbull. I figured he would be thrilled. He was.

And just in case they might be interested, I sent copies to the President of Jones University, the Dean of the Jones Law School, and the Dean of the Jones College of Arts and Sciences. Not being a vengeful person, I sent all this without comment.

But I did include copies of their 10-year-old letters turning Karen down.

So, you know, they could find the right file.

"Karen's going to 416, Dr. Galen," reports Natalie.

"Why is it, Natalie -- why is it -- that we may have three patients going into the hospital and you pick out Karen. For instance, you didn't tell me where Patton was going or where Treadway was going. Where are they going, by the way?"

"Patton's in 216 and Treadway's in ICU Blue."

"But mainly Karen's in 416, right?"

"Not exactly mainly. But, you know, she does get your attention."

"You mean, if you're also a young female."

'That's sort of sexist, Dr. Galen."

"Everybody has to have a sex."

"Well, nearly everybody."

"Like I said, Natalie --"

"Yessir?"

"How's the Xerox doing?"

131

INNER SANCTUM

I walk into the operating suite and check the Big Board for Jimmy Treadway. There it is: Pt Treadway, Surg Middleton, Rm 9.

Now you don't just *walk* into this sacred domain. I could just call Dr. Middleton on the intercom, interrupt him, ask him annoying questions. But it's better to show the proper respect. It's not necessary to actually genuflect, but the ritual is inviolable:

-change into scrub suit (daytime pajamas)

-put on the headgear (paper shower cap)

-cover your shoes (dainty booties with elastic top)

-scrub your hands and arms for at least 10 minutes with a brush and antiseptic soap, so as to remove the top layer of offending skin.

-don an outer robe of plastic-impregnated paper which ties in the back and hence cannot be used by anyone with bursitis.

-put on a cardboard mask which may or may not limit movement of bacteria but which does indeed retard movement of air into your lungs.

So far this is just to enter the room where the chosen are at work. If you're going to actually touch anything then you'll need to "double-glove" – a gymnastic task which only the initiated can perform without help. For me, the novitiate, the nurse must assist to assure that I don't contaminate the area.

"Dr Galen, how do you feel about Dr Lister's germ theory?" Joe Middleton asks across the operating table.

I suspect a trap. "Generally approve. Why?"

"You just scratched your nose with your glove."

"OK, I'll go back through the ritual. But is it permitted just to ask, How's the patient?"

"Fair. Ruptured spleen. Lacerated liver. Two tears in the bowel so far. We've fixed all that. A lot of bleeding. BP still 90 after 6 units. The potassium was still up – what was it, Maria?"

"It was 6.4, Dr. Middleton, let's see, 10 minutes ago."

I consider scratching my chin but hold off. "Guess we'll have to dialyze him right after surgery. Joe, can you put in a line we can use?"

"Already put in a triple-lumen in the left subclavian. Will that work?"

"Sure. Thanks. Guess I'll just take my germs and go back to the office."

The Treadway family sits in a tight knot, looking at the floor in the OR waiting room. All except for two: Larry the younger brother is asleep on his back under a chair and Harold, the older brother, is leaning against the wall in the corner eating a large piece of fried chicken. Again, they all get up when I walk in.

"Sit down, everybody, save your strength. Things are going about as well as we could hope so far." I tell about the spleen and the liver and the intestine, and explain about the artificial kidney.

133

"How can he live without a spleen?" asks Phyllis, one of the sisters. She has on a printed blouse which hangs outside her slacks.

"Well, the spleen mainly helps with infection, just like lymph nodes," I say. "We'll give him extra immunizations. People do OK without their spleen."

"Do you think he'll be able to ride tractors and horses again?" Asks Father Jack.

This is a code sentence. Jack can't bring himself to ask the more painful questions. Will Jimmy make it through surgery? Will he live through the day? Will he get out of this hospital? Instead he gives me a watered-down option.

"I'm afraid we're still at 50-50 right now. But things aren't any worse, and that's very good in this situation. Dr. Middleton will be out to talk with you after surgery – maybe in one or two hours."

Of course they always want to talk to the surgeon. He's been "in there." But then they'll want me again later, to ease the pain. Humankind, said Eliot, can only stand so much reality, or something like that.

THE BIG ONE

"I've never seen Roscoe Edwards like this," says Sandra, assuming her standard posture in the doorway: weight on left foot, right arm akimbo, right hip outthrust. "He's -- I don't know -- like a cat on a hot tin roof."

"I think he's worried," says Irene, sticking her head around the door, "Real worried."

"I really appreciate the psychosocial expertise I'm getting around here," I point out, "but all I actually want to know from you two is: What examining room is he in? And by the way, why the overpowering interest?"

They look at each other and giggle like teen-agers. Irene colors slightly. "He's cute."

I shake my head. "And what did he say was wrong with him?"

"That's it -- he didn't say," Sandra says. "That's always a sign of hidden anxiety."

"So you're psychiatrists, too. He won't hide the anxiety long. Probably wondering if he has gonorrhea. Or maybe AIDS. But, like I say, all I want to know is, What *room* is he in?"

"Number Four, Dr. Galen," says Irene. "Hope you'll tell us what the problem is."

"And private eyes, too. Don't you know about professional confidence? I can't tell you a damn' thing."

Roscoe Edwards is 27 and has always been healthy as a horse except for a little cardiac systolic murmur which we've studied and watched, but have generally felt quite sure is totally innocent. He does indeed look concerned sitting on his perch at the end of the examining table. His shirt is off and I notice wet spots on the roller paper where perspiration has dripped from his armpits.

"Hello, there, young feller. Looks like you've shed a few pounds."

"Yessir, twenty as a matter of fact."

"On purpose?"

135

"Oh, sure -- sticking to turnip greens and such. Got to get ready for the beach."

The chart shows 201 pounds last December and 179 today. "About 22, according to our scales, Roscoe. Wish everybody could do that on command. But what brings you in today, my friend?"

He sighes and flushes. He must now make the break and tell someone what's been causing him to wrestle with his pillow and with his imperfect knowledge -- probably for weeks. Why do people grovel in the pit of torment when they could simply ask a doctor? When he lets it out, whatever it is, he'll feel better, no matter what the outcome. At least his secretive pain will be tempered. He'll sleep through tonight, even if he does learn he has a venereal disease, or whatever.

"It's -- this, he says, pointing to the area just under his sternum. It's something growing there, and I guess you always think about cancer. I'm sick of worrying about it."

I have him lie flat on his back. Then I tell him to bring his knees up, in order to relax the rectus abdominis muscles and allow me to probe without resistance in his epigastric region, the spot directly above the navel. There, at the tip of the sternum, is a tail-like protuberance about one and one-half inches long. It is very hard. It is not tender. It tapers to a round point. It curls forward a little. It is clearly attached to the sternum itself.

"Is this what you mean, Roscoe?

He puts his finger next to mine. "Yes. Yessir. That's it. Is this the big one? Is it over?"

"Roscoe, it's not over. This is a nothing. Probably because you lost weight and therefore a little of your belly, you have unmasked and therefore discovered your xiphoid process."

"My *what?*"

"It's the tail of the sternum, or breastbone. Everybody has one. Some are like little knobs, some are like little fingers. Some are great long curvy hooks. They don't seem to have any evolutionary purpose since we came up to the two-footed stance, except to get young men scared to death when they find them. You're dismissed. I hope you never have anything worse."

I walk back to the office to try Mrs. Edison again. She called, said it was urgent, had to talk to me, then got on the line to someone else. Irene said she thinks the reason it's urgent is because Mrs. Edison she has to go to the beauty parlor. Line still busy.

"Well, Dr. Galen?"

"Oh, it's the local gossip columnists again."

"He looks relieved, Dr. Galen. What was it, what did you tell him?" Sandra again.

"Yeah, he's a new man," says Irene. "Even asked me about my new house when he came to get his insurance form."

"Well, it's not all that simple. He has, I'm afraid, a xiphoid process."

"A what?" Sandra.

"He said that too -- *What?*." I write *xiphoid process* down. "And there's no real treatment for it."

137

"Oh, God." Irene.

"I've told all of you -- you just can't get too emotionally involved in these patients. You'll pay the price."

They turn away, dejected.

Mean old doctor. But they're only twenty seconds away from *Stedman's Comprehensive Medical Dictionary*. Then *I'll* pay the price.

HUMORESQUE

I stand beside my desk, staring out the window over the parking lot into the trees, thinking of how we might improve Satchmo's situation, when Donna takes me by the hand and tugs me along.

"You've got to go see Mrs. Katzenberg right away. If you leave her in an examining room more than two minutes she starts yelling out and beating on the examining table with her umbrella."

"So that's my fault?"

"No, but you're just the only one who can bail us out. See her." Donna, of course, missed her big chance: in this day of feminine rights and with her natural equipment she could have, in the proper division of government, gone straight to field marshal.

Speaking of women, Mrs. Eleanor Katzenberg offers an interesting concatenation of characteristics. To begin with, she has always been an attractive, blue-eyed, rich, outspoken woman who qualifies, some would feel, as a Jewish American Princess. Certainly she behaves like a princess, demanding -- and almost always getting -- special concessions. Her

138

disposition has not improved with advancing age, diabetes, and hypertension, as well as with diet, Micronase, and Capoten. But so far it has always been possible to provoke a flash of secret delight in those pale blue eyes by offering her just the right bit of whimsy.

"What have you been doing with yourself, Mrs. K?"

"Nothing, of course. What can you do in my condition? If you were a better doctor maybe I could do something interesting."

"I was thinking maybe you'd been picking up some likely-looking men."

She looks toward the door, then back at me. She says, "Shit." Then she clasps her hand over her mouth, as if the expletive had just slipped out. But the eyes twinkle and we both know she has enunciated the word with far too much vituperation for any accident. Then, solemnly: "I don't pick up men." Eyes flash again: "They pick me up." The smile is now spreading: "If I can arrange it."

Her daughter Melody wonders at what she describes as "your patience in putting up with mother." But Melody is entrapped in the familiar mother-daughter guilt game which frequently evolves when loneliness and ill heath affect the parental figure: "Don't bother to come and see me this week. I know it's not very interesting over here. . . just because I haven't eaten in three days . . .If I get sick enough I'll just call the ambulance . . . or maybe the hearse. . . ." The daughter, usually the central family member who attends to mother's needs, is thereby injured, maybe even crushed.

Of course, Mrs. K tries to put the curse on me, too:

"I've been feeling terrible for a month."

"Why didn't you call me?"

"What, and be told you've gone skiing?"

"I don't go skiing in October."

"I can never get you."

"Everybody else does. Just yesterday about fifty people did."

"You can't help me, anyway."

Unlike the family member who is trapped, the physician must put up his shield here, recognize the patter of thinly veiled invective for what it is -- a plaint against life reaching its denouement -- and let it rain harmlessly off, much as the canvasback duck has learned to do. Otherwise he becomes defensive (and ineffective), angry (and frustrated), or, worse, is driven to put aside his standard chain of medical reasoning and make promises he can't keep -- thus compounding the disappointment which is such an integral part of life in this period of aging and loneliness.

The best solution is humor.

"Why don't you just call and leave word you have something interesting to tell me? Then I may rush and call you right back."

"I don't want to get you too excited, doctor."

"I need a little excitement in my life."

"OK, I'll call you every night."

Mrs. K's blood pressure and blood sugar prove to be 126/82 and 110, respectively: quite acceptable. She has no new findings on physical examination. We are checking the rest of her labwork.

"Let's keep on the same, except cut the captopril from 25 mgm to 12.5 mgm twice a day and we'll have the visiting nurse check your pressure several times. You're really doing pretty well, Eleanor. Don't you think so, Muriel?" I turn to the companion who always accompanies her everywhere.

Muriel is all smiles. "Yes, sir, she do just fine." Her eyes roll. "Most of the time."

"I don't do worth a shit and you both know it," says Eleanor. "And you"re not helping, doctor. I don't know why I come up here every three months. I'm not even well enough to make the trip."

"Too hard on you, Eleanor?" I ask.

"Sure is. Looks like somebody in my condition, you could come and make a house call."

"Just can't get here, eh, Eleanor? Well, tell me, how often do you go to the beauty parlor?"

"Oh, I don't know."

"What about that, Muriel?"

Muriel looks like Custer caught between two flanking bands of Indians. She looks right, then left at the galloping hordes. Then she smiles, and, like any good doomed soldier, faces her destiny.

"Oh, 'bout once, sometimes twice a week."

"What has the beauty operator got that I haven't, Eleanor?"

Eyes flash, grin spreads. "Lots." Eleanor says. "For one thing, he's bisexual. He can get twice as many dates as you."

Now she laughs aloud. Thank goodness.

141

ALTERED MENTAL STATUS

Irene walks in and plops a message in front of me. "Plops" is pretty accurate. Her body English says: *I know you don't want to be interrupted, but the floor nurse thinks this is important, and it's my job, so here it is, don't get mad at me, and if you do, I'm still doing what I have to and I'm not sorry. So there.*

Okay, okay, Irene. My irritated reactions to your messages are the reason for the plopping -- I'll try to do better. The management consultants for physicians' offices tell us the doctor is annoyed if he's interrupted or, later, will be annoyed if he wasn't. Moral: the personnel don't have a chance. This particular message says: Mrs. Jones in Room 537 is not doing well, trying to get up and go home, thinks the police are after her, says the orderly is a burglar. She was hard to arouse this morning, did you wake her up on rounds, Doctor?

"Irene?" Where is Irene now? "Irene, come back here please." Wrong button on the intercom. Ruth says: "Not here, sorry." Next button. "IRENE!" She appears. "Irene, please get the nurse on the line about Mrs. Jones."

Sandra comes in with a raft of prescription refills. "More homework." She gives me a glowing smile, don't know how she can always work up a glowing smile over prescription refills. I can't work up a smile over anything right now.

"IRENE! Did you get --"

"Juanita is on the phone about Mrs. Jones, Dr. Galen." Irene's voice over the intercom sounds like it's coming from the bottom of a dry well.

"Juanita?"

"Yes, Dr. Galen."

"Sounds like Mrs. Jones has lost her cool over there."

"Yes, sir, she was okay last night, maybe a little jumpy. But she's definitely out of her tree right now."

"I'll be there shortly. Meanwhile, let's check blood gases, SMA-6 stat, SMA-12 ASAP. Does she seem short of breath or anything?"

"Not particularly. Or . . . no more than usual. Respirations about 24, but that's par for her."

"Better get a quick saturation with the oximeter, too. Thanks." I hang up, walk around to check on the chest film on Mrs. Flaherty in Room 3, tell Sandra to warn the other patients I've got to go to the hospital on an emergency, give Mrs. Flaherty a prescription for her bronchitis ("No pneumonia, Mrs. F., I'm glad to say"), and sneak out the back door, the wonderful secret exit. You always have to tell patients it's an emergency when you do something to keep them waiting. If they sit at length with no explanation, they become irritated. If someone is apparently taken out of turn, they get irate. If they think they're forgotten, they act desperate. If, on the other hand, you explain you have an emergency, all is forgiven ("Sorry I kept you waiting, Mr. Sanderson." "Oh, no, no problem, Dr. Galen -- I'd want you to come to me if *I* had an emergency.") You don't tell them that sometimes it wasn't that important, just a matter of

143

getting the emergency room nurse off your back. The surgeons have a better excuse: they are, whenever it's convenient, "tied up in the operating room." This expression gives me visions of gown-clad men and women gagged and bound in the corner of the sterile suite, struggling vainly with their bonds. It exempts them from unwanted telephone calls, meetings, office patients, nagging internists. I've often considered protesting that I'm "tied up with the artificial kidney." But people know too much nowadays: the nurse does most of that and anyway it's not dramatic enough. How about "tied up in meditation over this last case"?

That won't fly either.

The elevators seem to have been warned I was coming and have left on coffee break. The more pressed I am, the longer they take, and then they'll stop on every floor. Finally, we arrive at 5-South and I walk the long corridor down to 5-North. In 537 Mrs. Jones is roiling around in her bed with a vacant expression. At age 67 she came in with acute bronchitis which, superimposed on her chronic obstructive lung disease (a modernism for emphysema), put her into a fairly severe attack of pulmonary insufficiency. That is, her lungs, already short of the standard exchange rate for oxygen and carbon dioxide, got worse. Ordinarily, the brain stem and the respiratory apparatus jealously guard the balance of these blood gas levels. Measured in millimeters of mercury, normal values are rigidly enforced at the 35 to 45 mm Hg level for carbon dioxide partial pressure ("pCO2") and 75-85 mm Hg for oxygen ("pO2"). If your lungs flag in their duty of getting in the precious oxygen and getting out the waste product CO_2, you feel short of breath and you just don't do well; you might even get branded as a *chronic lunger*. Cora Jones' day-to-day values are, typically, 48 for pCO_2 and 55-60 for pO_2 -- markedly impaired. When she came into the emergency room five days ago, the numbers were considerably worse: pCO_2 58 and pO_2 42. The interns say irreverently (they are always irreverent, it lessens the pain) that anyone with these numbers is a member of the "50-50 Club." She was cyanotic (that's medical code for *blue*), she was struggling for breath, her lungs were full of wheezes, and she had Impending Doom written all over her. Well she might: one of her most basic functions -- gas exchange -- was on the blink. She responded, as most do, to a combination of oxygen by positive-pressure mask, terbutaline by inhalation (to open up the bronchial tubes), methylprednisolone (to reduce inflammation in the respiratory tract), and antibiotics. She seemed to be resting comfortably when I looked in this morning, but she's not comfortable now.

"Doctor Simpson," she calls out, referring to her previous family practitioner, now retired, "I'm sick -- take me to the hospital!"

I explain that's where she is, I'm Dr. Galen, she'll be all right.

She is not reassured.

"These people keep coming in my windows and trying to take me to jail," she exclaims. She has now been restrained, with a decidedly unstylish if effective Posey belt around her middle and a wrist restraint on the arm with the IV

145

going -- neither garment available at Neiman-Marcus. She struggles with both of her canvas shackles.

"Any word on the lab yet, Juanita?"

"Not yet, but I'll call them, Dr. Galen." She leaves to go to the nursing station phone, knowing that the computer, vaunted for its speed by its enthusiastic young pin-striped purveyors, will be the last to know, particularly in an urgent situation. Only real people, concerned for the welfare of other real people, will break through the carefully rigged but bureaucratic information chain to get results before the printout surfaces or the screen lights up.

Meanwhile, I examine Mrs. Jones, looking for clues to her confusional state. Now, if you are a Doctor, and if you are concerned about your status among your peers, you must be aware of proper terminology. Years ago you would call Mrs. Jones' present problem "acute organic brain syndrome." Then, more recently, "acute encephalopathy." Now, if you are *au courant,* you will blithely intone the phrase "Altered Mental State," or, if you are as *de rigueur* as the medical residents, "AMS." All the terms mean the same thing: the patient is out to lunch and we don't know why, but we'd better find out quick.

To find out, you have to consider a lot of potential causes for this sudden change of a human being's mentation. First of all, as in Mrs. Jones' case, you know it's not a psychological quirk: regular hysteria or schizophrenia or paranoia aren't normally associated with a loss of the intellectual perception of one's surroundings. Patients with a purely emotional break generally know where they are, who

146

they are, who you are, what day it is, etc. That is, they are "oriented" (I've always wondered if, in Bejing, you are "occidented").

Mrs. Jones can't make it on any of these scores. Her intellectual machinery is in an acute state of disarray. So we have to consider a whole list of other possibilities responsible for this organic dysfunction. First, her lung status may have deteriorated. Her oxygen may have gone back down or her CO_2 may have climbed: either will cause the brain to misfire. Kidneys can stop doing their job of purifying the blood of metabolic wastes and uremia can result. Blood electrolytes (the standard label for minerals) could be out of whack. Maybe drugs have caused this, or even -- as sometimes happens -- drug withdrawal. If the liver decompensates, mental changes follow. Thyroid or adrenal problems can do it. Over-whelming infection -- "sepsis" -- causes the brain to go awry.

Older people -- Mrs. Jones at only 67 seems fairly young to me these days -- will sometimes get confused in the hospital and no one really knows why. Often this happens just at twilight: they are said to "sundown." The typical patient, perhaps a man of 80, is recovering well from his fractured hip and discusses politics with the floor nurses at 11 a. m. At 6 p. m., however, dusk sets in and he wants to get a cab back to Brooklyn so he can finish those tax papers. When you won't let him up he gets agitated, reveals unsuspected strength, and has to be sedated with Vistaril or Thorazine for days; then, abruptly, he recovers.

In other cases -- for example, renal patients who are approaching dialysis -- a peculiar picture like acute schizophrenia emerges. In the morning you note only that the patient has a fast pulse and seems more vigilant than usual. That afternoon he is strangely euphoric. The next day he smiles confidently and tells you that everything is fine now. He has a direct pipeline to God and can control the world around him through the simple expedient of manipulating his own thoughts. Later that day he withdraws from the world. His lids are closed. Although his vital signs are normal, he won't speak or open his eyes. He may exhibit the stiffness, the "waxy flexibility," of catatonia. The blood chemistries have showed no change. The psychiatrist is unable to get any past history of weird behavior from the family. Here again, the patient must be given phenothiazines or similar drugs and watched closely. To everyone's surprise, this seemingly terminal deterioration evaporates within three to five days and our subject returns to his previous status, usually blithely innocent of the whole affair. I've seen this sufficiently often now to be able to reassure family and other physicians that "everything will be all right soon." They are generally skeptical but later on you gain a little more credibility; you may even gain a little respect.

Now, examining Mrs. Jones, I find no clues. I realize that we must have help from the lab, and I ponder upon the rapidity with which we have become dependent on chemical analysis in our day-to-day practice. Many blood chemistries, such as sodium and potassium levels, in my father's time were almost a research procedure; now they are available in an hour. In my son's day these and many more values will probably appear as the patient comes through the door. A sensor mounted in the ceiling of the reception room will probably instantly perceive total body zinc, scan the genome, count the proteins and project it all on a screen.

Well, anyway, here comes Juanita. With a sheet of paper. "Gases are OK. The only big glitch is her sodium, Dr. Galen. It's 115."

I know -- and so does Juanita -- that this number is way off, the normal value for sodium concentration being 135-145 milliequivalents per liter. And I also know that an abrupt drop in the salt level will cause anything from slight mental haziness to coma and convulsions. Now we'll have to figure out why this happened and correct it -- and the trick is, with low-sodium syndromes, things are frequently not what they seem. You might naturally presume that a low salt level means salt deficiency -- so therefore you need to give the patient a lot of salt pronto. But then you would be using ordinary logic, and this is not ordinary logic, it's human biology. Strangely, in the hospitalized patient, a very low sodium in the blood more often than not means, not too little sodium, but too much water.

It was only some thirty years ago that a former mentor of mine discovered this. This man, Bill Blackman, through no special fault of his own, was (and is) a natural-born genius: he didn't (and doesn't) think quite like other people. He was able to puzzle out the fact that in a wide variety of medical conditions the pituitary gland gets the notion to keep making its water-retaining hormone (antidiuretic hormone

149

[ADH]) when it's not needed. The result, of course, is that too much water accumulates in the body. Then, for some bizarre reason, the kidneys, restricted in their ability to dump water, decide to dump sodium instead. Thus, the sodium concentration in the blood, already lowered by dilution, is lowered further. Treatment? Restrict water, otherwise the trend will keep getting worse, no matter how much salt you pour in.

Bill Blackman's hypothesis, brainstorm that it was, received short shrift from his peers at the time. I remember well his description to a group of us fellows-in-training sitting around the lab at the Northeast Medical Center some years later. Bill had presented his findings to the Kidney and Electrolyte crowd at National Institutes of Health in Bethesda, he told us. In that group were the leading lights in the blood mineral business and one by one they discouraged him. One international metabolic wizard said he didn't know what those cases meant; another researcher with an IQ of about 180 and a propensity to offer acerbic comments, said he didn't either but doubted the ADH thing. A third renal authority, later to become editor of a national medical journal, suggested that it might be some strange form of adrenal insufficiency. Only Frank Buyer, wily guru of the Metabolic Section, puffed on his pipe and nodded his white head knowingly. Nowadays, since their first skeptically received article in a major medical journal in 1957, "The Syndrome of Sustained, Inappropriate Secretion of Antidiuretic Hormone (SIADH)" -- or the "Blackman-Buyer Syndrome" -- has become a fixture in medical thinking. Later, more sophisticated technology has made it possible actually to measure the amount of the hormone in the blood.. As of 2003, a computer-directed Medline search of the world literature on the syndrome – originally doubted -- revealed over seventeen hundred articles. Yet even now, many physicians seem unaware of this entity, or have heard of it and don't understand it. Every week or so I find myself outlining the physiologic basis to physicians whose eyes say they don't exactly believe -- or don't exactly follow -- the explanation . . . of a clinical disturbance which is now three decades old.

I recall the court scene not too long ago. It was a malpractice case in which a doctor was accused of giving too much water to a young patient with a kidney stone. As she lapsed into stupor she was shipped from her rural hospital setting to a medical center, where her sodium was found to have plummeted to 118 meq/L. But even the sophisticated physicians at the university hospital -- four of them -- failed to tip to the key fact: she had suddenly developed SIADH then recovered. Her country doctor wasn't at fault: human biology had erred again.

Explaining this to a lay jury in the courthouse in the middle of a tiny rural village was quite a challenge. But after I brought in a transparent plastic bucket half full of tinted salt-water and then added plain water -- much to the chagrin of the plaintiff's attorney -- you could see the heads nodding in understanding. When they acquitted the doctor, I figured I had accomplished a tour-de-force. Then I learned that the discussion in the jury room had climaxed with a white-haired lady telling the hold-out juror, "Ruby, that there city doctor said everything was all right, so just vote 'Not guilty.'" She did. (And still later they told me that it had taken 3 years to find jurors who didn't think the accused doctor had saved their lives.)

The patient, by the way, is doing fine. It was interesting to me that none of the lawyers at the original deposition before the trial knew her present condition when I asked. These lawyers, I guess, are contemporary cowboys desperately struggling to avenge her experience through the modern equivalent of a confrontation on the main street of old Abilene -- legal and fiscal violence. Only her doctor -- the one she was suing -- responded: "Susie's doing OK, he said. "I see her on the street and ask about her. She says she has no complaints. Doing pretty good in school, playing basketball."

Maybe the quizzical doctors at my hospital and those at the medical center are today's counterpart of Blackman's and Buyer's dubious peers. Anyway, good work, Bill and Frank. And good work, little country jury.

And thanks to all of those, because now I believe that's what Mrs. Jones has. Not any of the many other causes of low sodium -- like dehydration from vomiting and diarrhea, or diuretics, or adrenal insufficiency. Not the dislocation that may occur with congestive heart failure or liver failure or other edema states.

But SIADH. She has the clues: she has no signs of dehydration, she has a background of obstructive lung disease (one of the many conditions which can bring on SIADH), and I just bet she has a lot of sodium in her urine. We'll see. Meanwhile, we'll restrict water and give her a little concentrated salt solution, just enough to boost her back toward reality.

"Let's grab a urine specimen for sodium, Juanita. And put her on NPO. Hang 500 ml of 3% saline. Start it at 100 ml per hour, please, ma'am. I think she has SIADH."

"All right, Dr. Galen." Juanita is jotting and moving at the same time. She jogs to the nursing station, calls the pharmacy, tells the ward clerk to feed the order into the computer. Then, her tasks well under way for the moment, she turns to me as I'm writing on the order sheet.

"And you said that was S - I - what?"

"SIADH. Syndrome of Inappropriate Anti-Diuretic Hormone Secretion."

"How did she get it?"

"A lot of sick people develop it. Especially pulmonary patients. It was discovered about thirty years ago."

"Oh. That's older than I am. But I never heard of it."

"Well, I'll tell you about it when we both get a break sometime soon."

"Thanks a lot, Dr. Galen. That'll be great. I guess I'm the only one who doesn't know about it."

"No, Juanita, you're not the only one."

PAIN OF UNKNOWN ORIGIN

"Jan is on the phone, Dr. Galen--you know, the ER nurse." Sandra looks as if she knows something I don't.

She does. "You know, you're on call for the emergency room today."

Oh, God. Twenty-four hours of being the bail-out man, the one who takes hospital admissions of those patients who don't have a regular doctor. Sometimes the dreaded period goes by quietly, even without your realizing you were "in the barrel"; at other times, it may bring three or four admissions -- often tough cases. And commonly "no pay."

I punch the button with the glittering light. The light goes out and Julie Higgins comes on. She's the cute, sassy one.

"Young man with abdominal pain, Dr. Galen. Acts like a kidney stone, but the ER doctor, Dr. Anders, ordered a spiral CT scan and it's negative. Urine negative. CBC and SMA-6 negative. So it's abdominal pain, cause unknown. We think we need a Real Doctor."

"Know any?"

"Sure, that's why we dialed this number. The rotofile says 'John Galen, RD.'"

"What about the yellow pages?"

"Haven't looked there. Probably just says MD, internal medicine and nephrology."

"Not ER consultant?"

"Nope. Want me to have them add that?"

"Lord, no. See you in a few minutes."

COMPLAINTS AND CODES

Dan Godwick is a 24-year-old State Tech student who is now writhing in pain on the stretcher in Room 4 of the emergency suite. He is holding his right flank.

I introduce myself and ask when the pain started.

154

"About 4 o'clock this morning, Doctor. It's getting worse."

"Does it come and go, or is it steady?" I know that a kidney, or ureteral, stone, characteristically produces an intense pain which builds up, then lets off, rather than a continuous one, though it may be of either type.

"Steady. It doesn't stop." Dan tells me he's had two stones in the past and just two weeks ago was hospitalized in Little Rock, Arkansas, where a urologist did a retrograde study (that's using a cystoscope and going up through the penis) and "pushed a stone back up from the ureter into the kidney."

"Funny it doesn't show now on the X-ray," I offer.

"It didn't then. That's why they had to do the retrograde."

"Oh." I reflect that some stones -- about 15% -- aren't visible on X-Ray. These are usually made of uric acid instead of the more common calcium oxalate. I examine Dan and find his abdominal muscles tense but when he breathes deeply or is distracted, they relax. He is not really tender on the right side where he hurts. There are no lumps or masses. His bowel sounds seem normal. The cause of his abdominal pain remains a mystery so far, but intense pain without guarding or objective tenderness is quite compatible with a stone in the urinary tract; appendicitis -- the common and most immediate concern -- is unlikely.

"We'd better admit you and do more tests," I suggest. "If the pain doesn't resolve right away, we may have to check

155

out your gallbladder, rule out an ulcer. We may even have to do another retrograde."

"OK, Doctor. Can I have something for this pain?"

"Sure." The emergency room physician hadn't prescribed pain medication yet – not from callousness but from obeying the general medical policy never to give analgesics to a patient with abdominal pain until the responsible physician has seen him: the nature of the problem may be masked for hours until the drug wears off. I now order an injection containing Demerol for pain and Phenergan for nausea and request hospital admission. Then I write orders for management, including intravenous fluids and instructions to keep him fasting. In the doctor-nurse code, that's NPO (*nil per os* --nothing by mouth).

It occurs to me that it's *nice* to have a code, makes you feel important. Particularly since we doctors have lost a lot of our secret language in recent years: we hardly use Latin anymore, don't use the good old archaic symbols, even write so people can read it sometimes. Patients have copies of the PDR (Physicians' Desk Reference) at home, look up things on the internet, ask you about the side effects and contraindications. It takes away from the magic.

Of course, we still cling to a few clandestine phrases to sustain our sense of exclusivity. We write SOB for Shortness of Breath (and maybe get rid of a trace of hostility in the process). PTA has nothing to do with grade school --it means Prior To Admission. WDWNWF is a Well-Developed, Well-Nourished White Female. BRBPR is even used for Bright Red Bleeding Per Rectum. The phrase ac

156

(*ante cibum*) signifies before meals. But this alphabetization is a far cry from the elegant Latin of Sir William Osler, with *materia medica* and *aequinimitas* tripping off the tongue and flowing from the pen.

Even in my dad's day a prescription for a routine cold pill had all the proper hieroglyphics of a wizard's potion:

Acetyl-salicylic acid	gr v
Acetaminophen	gr v
Pseudo-ephedrine	
Codeine sulfate	gr 1/4
M & Disp # 24	
Sig: i – ii q4h prn for pain and discomfort	

_____MD

Now you'd just write for "Vicodin" and have them pick up an across-the-counter decongestant. The patient knows all about antibiotics, aspirin, and codeine, knows if she can or can't tolerate them. The mystery -- and with it the mastery -- is gone. Now all I'm left with is codes like NPO. So I write it with just a little flourish.

Thus far I've relied mostly on clinical assessment to handle Dan's problem. If he's is not better by midday, I figure, we'll break down and resort to modern diagnostic technology.

CAMPY DIAGNOSES

Sandra shows Gloria Branham into my office and into the burnt-orange leather chair opposite my desk. In Suite 350, if you're a new patient, you get to come into the office first. If you're an old patient you usually are shuttled, some think unceremoniously, into an examining room and told to strip garments away from suspicious areas. But this is the first visit for Gloria, so she gets the office and the burnt-orange leather chair.

The value of this process of talking -- or "taking a history" -- has been much underestimated in recent years. In this grotesquely technological era people expect quick answers from magic machines. They want a computer printout telling them they don't have cancer; they demand a synthesized image showing the cause of the pain. "Did the EKG show the cause of this chest tightness?" or "I couldn't have a stroke with a normal cholesterol, could I?" or "You say I have migraine but shouldn't I have a CAT scan to confirm it?" are common protestations in our office. It's hard to get across the message to most people (and we don't know yet if Gloria is one of them) that the crucial diagnostic information is usually obtained in the historical interview. After all, the patient is the only machine equipped with a series of continuous sensing mechanisms of all body systems. The only device provided with a million nerves ramifying to every nook and cranny of Gloria's body -- is Gloria. She is her own round-the-clock private duty nurse, she is her own continuous monitor. Sir William Osler, father of modern medicine (and now -- erroneously -- judged by some to be outdated in his turn-of-century concepts) said "If you listen to the patient long enough, he'll tell you what's wrong with him." It is still true that 85% of the diagnosis lies in the patient's description of symptoms. The students and house

158

officers think of me as a broken (and probably obsolescent 75-rpm) record on this point: "If you haven't found the answer after the history and physical," I keep saying, "it's not time to turn to the scanner or the SMA machines. It's time to take another history." Joan Rivers has the right phrase: "Can we talk?"

Something, though, tells me that Gloria Burnham isn't going to take to this hypothesis very well. Maybe it's the way she begins her recitation of problems:

"I was diagnosed with hypoglycemia ten years ago. I was put on treatment by a wonderful doctor and felt so much better. Then in the last year I've just felt terrible and it's taken all this time to find out I have chronic Epstein-Barr virus. Nothing has done any good and so that's why I'm here." She smiles, rather engagingly. "Are you good at treating these diseases?"

My biggest problem is to hide the sigh. "Well, we'll see, we'll certainly do our best."

But I'm afraid I have already seen . . . that Gloria is probably the unfortunate victim of the growing tendency to take vague symptoms and tag them with a charismatic diagnostic label. And the diagnostic labels are more dubious than the symptoms. So here we are: a large number of people are walking our planet suffering from *non-diseases*.

I ask Gloria to go back and give me the details of her experiences.

"Well, when I first started with hypoglycemia (she's still giving me diagnoses), I felt weak and run-down all the time and would have to eat constantly to feel better. I gained weight and got worse and worse."

"Did you have spells of weakness, shakiness, perspiration? Did they come on with relation to your meals?"

"Well, yes. Sometimes. But I just felt bad all the time. I would cry a lot, couldn't get anything done, felt hopeless. Hated to get up in the morning. The nights were terrible. I would wake up at 3 o'clock in the morning and couldn't go back to sleep. My friends said I had a hang-dog look. And all the time I had hypoglycemia and didn't know it."

"Gloria, I presume the doctor put you on a diet when he diagnosed (note I don't say discovered) the hypoglycemia."

"Yes. No sweets. Up till that time I had been eating candy bars right and left, trying to combat my bad feelings. He said it made things worse, I needed to be on a low carbohydrate diet, not a high one."

"And then you got better?"

"Not right away. But over a few weeks I began to feel better. I lost some weight. But I still didn't get back to normal. Then I joined the Consortium."

"The Consortium? "

"Yes. The Hypoglycemia Consortium. It's a national organization, dedicated to the relief of hypoglycemia sufferers. They have literature, support groups. Oh, gosh, that scares me -- don't tell me you don't *know* about it."

"Oh, yes, I know about it." And indeed I do. Early in my practice, I wrote off for material from this group. Two weeks later I received what can only be described as a shipment: five pounds of pamphlets, almost exclusively written and/or prepared by lay "experts" on hypoglycemia. The material went into great detail about the symptoms, and well it might, for these are virtually all the symptoms which afflict mankind:

--- headache, weakness, blurry vision, ears ringing, neck stiffness, chest tightness, shortness of breath tingling in the extremities, heartburn, abdominal pain, indigestion, urinary frequency, ad infinitum . . .

. . . and all ascribed to, you guessed it, the menacing phenomenon of hypoglycemia. The Consortium people were careful to point out that most doctors don't even *know* about this: "You must find a doctor who's a hypoglycemia specialist, or you may go through life suffering needlessly." They also laid out the diagnostic essentials: "A five-hour, or even eight-hour, glucose tolerance test must be done, or it will be missed. A slight drop in the blood sugar, of a degree usually dismissed by doctors, is significant."

The devotees of this condition are legion: they lead and populate the support groups; there are psychiatric social workers who love the entity; each newspaper has at least one feature writer who is a card-carrying member, if not of the Consortium, at least of the Movement. You can't blame them. It's easy to see how the trap can spring and ensnare them: here, after all, is a way to explain the vast spectrum of human suffering, and the panacea is just a diet!

161

It occurs to me that Gloria is a marvelous demonstration case, able to capsule a famous diagnostic category into a few sentences. But the famous category she typifies isn't hypoglycemia; it's the far more common, far more real, far more devastating one of psychic depression. The educational process, including deprogramming her from her misconceptions and redirecting her to reality, will take a long time, and I'm not even ready to begin yet, because *she* isn't ready.

But the facts are, these good people are misled. Not that hypoglycemia, or low blood sugar, is non-existent. It's just not a big public health hazard, and for most people, like Gloria, it's not the problem. Indeed, all of the fad diagnoses have some truth behind them: that's what makes a doctor's life difficult. There *is* an EB Virus, there *is* a Temporomandibular Joint Syndrome, there *is* such a thing as Mitral Valve Prolapse, there *is* a Premenstrual Syndrome. But they don't explain all the mysteries -- and the miseries -- of life.

Hypoglycemia, for example, comes in three forms. The first is that seen in diabetics taking insulin. Then there is "organic" hypoglycemia, due to a tumor of the pancreas which produces insulin ("beta-cell adenoma"). Removal of the tumor cures them. But this is a rare bird: I've only seen three in twenty-five years.

And then -- here is the big problem -- reactive hypoglycemia. When you eat a meal containing a certain amount of carbohydrate, or eat a candy bar, your blood sugar rises, then falls. The rise, clearly, is due to the absorption of glucose; the fall is due to the insulin your pancreas produces in response to the glucose. This hormone drives the sugar into your tissues, out of the bloodstream. Sometimes the level falls below the original fasting value. Occasionally, if the drop is fast enough, it may trigger efforts to compensate: your sympathetic nervous system is stimulated, your adrenal glands are turned on, you feel shaky, weak, sweaty. Almost everybody has experienced this at some time: eat pancakes with syrup on an empty stomach, and two hours later you're a basket case. You can cure this with a sweet soft drink or orange juice.

Or you can wait a few minutes for your body to readjust. People who customarily eat a lot of sugar "rev up" their pancreatic insulin factory to such a degree that this drop occurs all the time. These are the ones who can benefit from a no-sweet, low-carbohydrate diet which "detunes" their beta cells. But it's important to point out that they are annoyed by this phenomenon; they are not disabled by it, as some would suggest.

Even dogs can be made to exhibit this trend. I remember well when I first learned this as a freshman medical student. I couldn't wait to spring it on my physician-father (who then was a dinosaur of twenty-five years' practice-- *and what am I now – after 30 years?*).

"Dad, I bet you can't tell me what happens when you give a dog high-carbohydrate feedings for a month."

No answer.

I kept on. "What will his glucose-tolerance curve look like?"

Silence. He was moving toward the desk in the bedroom. Probably going to try to look it up.

I persisted further. "Will his postabsorption blood sugar be higher or lower?"

His tall, angular figure, topped by the thinning, wavy red hair, had now reached the desk, and he was digging in the bottom right-hand drawer.

"Well, I understand," I told him, chortling. "You can't be expected to keep up with everything."

Then he came up with a piece of printed material and handed it to me. It was a yellowed though well-preserved reprint of an article from the Southern Medical Journal, dated 1931 (the same year Banting and Best discovered insulin). This article described the treatment of reactive hypoglycemia in humans with a high-protein, high-fat, low carbohydrate diet. Several cases were well presented, the physiology was discussed in some detail, and the beneficial results of the proposed dietary program were outlined. The article systematically reviewed the world literature up to that point and, in the process, referred to some of the previous experimental data in dogs and other species that I had cited.

It was the first clinical report of use of such a diet in the treatment of reactive hypoglycemia. It was written by a single author.

My father.

Dealing with Gloria's perception of the Epstein-Barr thing is going to be harder than recovering from my father's *coup*. The EB virus is the known cause of infectious mononucleosis, or "mono," a common disease among adolescents. Because of the suspected transmission via saliva, it is often referred to as the "kissing disease." It causes sore throat, enlarged lymph nodes, loss of appetite, and a characteristic malaise, or fatigue. It lasts, usually, about three weeks, and the sufferer ordinarily feels tired for another fortnight or so.

Overpowering lassitude may be responsible for this favorite medical hallucination. Since so many people have, or complain of, chronic fatigue, lethargy, lack of energy, it was perhaps inevitable that someone would conceive of a chronic mono state, draw a blood test for antibodies, find it high, and, eureka, discover a new syndrome. Problem is, anybody who has had mono at any time -- or even been exposed to it -- has these antibodies, sometimes in high titers. The Harvard Medical Letter, that excellent publication for the lay audience, has laid the matter to rest thus: "There may be many explanations for the chronic fatigue syndrome, but chronic infection with the EB virus is not one of them." So, no magic explanation for fatigue here. Just as there was none in the era of "chronic brucellosis," or "soldier's heart," or "chronic neurasthenia". Gloria and I will have to have a long talk later.

It takes a lot longer to unmake a diagnosis than to make one.

Like hypoglycemia, the premenstrual syndrome (PMS) has found an extensive following. And, like low-blood sugar, it has some fragments of a physiological basis. Everyone knows that hormonal fluctuations occur in the female menstrual cycle: estrogen rises to a peak right before the period, then plummets. Meanwhile progesterone builds up before and during the period. This interface of hormonal changes cause the menstrual flow to occur. There are other effects, too: high estrogen can cause fluid retention, a little irritability, sometimes headache. Often diuretics and agents to control menstrual cramps are useful. But a vast delusion has now built up -- certain women complain they are premenstrual for two weeks or even *all the time.* PMS Clinics have sprung up. Fascinating formulations are recommended or even prescribed: pyridoxine, vitamin E, magnesium -- all generally harmless but also irrational and without proven benefit. In Britain, a court dismissed two women of a murder charge because they "weren't responsible for their actions" -- they were in the middle of PMS!

Now, mitral valve prolapse (MVP) is another whole ball game. I'm thinking of starting a support group for people who *don't have* MVP. After all, they are greatly limited in their conversation at the beauty parlor or on the golf course. They are victims of social deprivation. They deserve help.

MVP consists of a tendency of one of the heart valves to balloon upwards when the biggest chamber (the left ventricle) contracts. This event makes a little sound the doctor can hear with the stethoscope, called an "ejection click." The sound tends to come and go and is made more obvious by having the patient stand. A device known as the echocardiogram (similar to a sonar fish-finder) may show the valve flopping, or it may not.

That's all most people with MVP have -- a click. In some, the valve bulges upward enough for the leaflets to drop apart, and they have a murmur -- meaning there is a little regugitant jet of blood going backwards from the left ventricle into the left atrium. We usually give those with a murmur antibiotics for dental work.

More disabling is the notion that the very common condition of mitral valve prolapse (10-20% of women and 5-6% of men) makes you somehow ill. You're supposed to have (1) episodes of atypical chest pain. You're expected to (2) drop your blood pressure when you stand. You're more (3) nervous, are subject to episodes of (4) palpitation and (5) hyperventilation. It's very convenient for the doctor to be able to blame all these symptoms on MVP. But what about all those people without MVP who regularly report symptoms 1 through 5?

If a person, a woman, say, has a click and/or murmur, she is eligible to join the Club -- and be popular at the supermarket social or the cocktail party. True, she should ask her doctor about prophylactic antibiotics. But she shouldn't put herself on the injured list!

Fortunately, people have a basic skepticism, they become inured to hollow rhetoric, and, perhaps more important, they tire easily of new fads. Thus PMS will pass into obscurity eventually. Chronic fatigue syndrome will pall after a sufficient number of headlines. Hypoglycemia has done this already several times, only to re-emerge as new generations encounter again the hyperbole of the press, the desperation produced by anxiety, and the inadequately bridled enthusiasm of uncritical therapeuticians.

There are plenty of other non-diseases, but it's time to move on.

HOUSE CALL

I pick up the next telephone message. Madison Hartwell wants me to make a house call on his wife today. She is sick with cough, chest pain, and high fever, and doesn't feel like coming to the office.

I call Madison and carefully *do not* tell him it would destroy my -- and my patients' -- day to leave the clinic and hospital to ride through traffic at high noon. I also leave out the part about the high overhead and needing to stay in business so I can continue to be his family doctor, etc.

What I *do* tell him is also true and is a little more palatable.

"Madison, it sounds a lot like pneumonia, and I know we'll have to get a chest x-ray to be sure we get Agnes on the right treatment. We can't do that at home. If you can bring her to the office we'll get her in right away and take care of it. If she's too sick to ride in the car, call an ambulance and get her to the emergency room. Either way, we'll get her what she needs."

"Just a minute, John."

I hear conversation in the background.

"We insist you come out, John. After you examine her, you can decide if an ambulance is necessary."

168

"OK, Madison. I'll come out. But as I say, I already know we'll have to bring her in for a film."

"Wait another second."

"OK."

"She says she'll come in the car."

"Fine. I'll alert the front desk. Shall we send a wheelchair down to the building entrance so you can wheel her up?

"Well, no, John, I - I - guess I won't be coming with her. She should be able to drive OK."

"Oh."

"You know how it is, John."

"How's that, Madison?"

"I'm sure you'll understand -- one of the things you just can't do is let your foursome down."

But house calls are absolutely invaluable. And fun. They are worth the effort and the lost revenue. You learn things that you could never discover any other way. The wife is waited on hand and foot by the husband, who seems to ask permission even to go to the bathroom. The elderly lady, bedridden with Parkinsonism and who is the matron of a very wealthy family, stays awake all night watching videos, then sleeps all day and won't eat. That is, until I have a conversation with her about nasogastric tube feedings and intravenous alimentation, after which interview she becomes strangely ravenous. Furthermore I learn that 3 a.m. is the time when she asks the private-duty nurse to put on the triple-x rated film, and that she laughs through the whole thing.

169

Another well-to-do widow, with an average of three staff hovering over her at any given time, insists on my making monthly house calls because ever since her hip fracture she's not mobile. After a year and about 8 visits, I urge a trip to the office for lab tests and X-Rays.

"John, you know I just can't get out with this hip," says Victoria.

On the way out, I turn to the companion. Does Mrs. Smythe never get out of the house?"

"Oh, yessir, she get out."

"How often?"

"Oh, 'bout once a week."

"Really? Where does she go?"

"To her chiropractor."

But the most revealing of all unscheduled out-of-office experiences involved Mrs. Levinson. Mrs. L was a long-term patient, ensconced in a very nice local nursing home. Though 94, she was frankly brilliant, amazingly informed, and a conversational whiz. No visit to her bedside was complete without a roundup on the political scene and, perhaps, Tolstoy's view of the world. I got a midnight call saying that Mrs. L, by now a mere wraith, had been badly injured by a confused resident named Mrs. Genevieve Highsmith who had come into Mrs. L's room by wheelchair and simply beat her up.

I rushed out, examined Mrs L, ordered X-rays, and concluded that luckily we were only dealing with scrapes and bruises. I advised the staff to do something about the

170

demented attacker, since she had now become dangerous, and I was assured she would be moved to the Alzheimer Unit.

Mrs. L died from complications of her chronic lung disease about a year later and, to please the family and myself, I journeyed out to pronounce her. It was then I learned something more about the incident. The charge nurse was the one to tell me.

"That was really something about Mrs Levinson getting beat up by Mrs Highsmith," said Nurse Joan Johanssen.

"Yes, too bad . . . for both of them."

"Well, you know how it happened."

"How do you mean?"

"Mrs. Highsmith was wheeling around the ward the way she always did."

"Yes?"

"And went into Mrs. Levinson's room. Mrs. L said, 'Genevieve, do you know what I've got under this sheet?' She pointed to a couple of pillows she had put under the covers. Mrs. Highsmith said, 'No, what?'

"'It's your husband.' And that's when Mrs. Levinson got beat up."

A TESTING SITUATION

At noon, Dan Godwick is no better. The floor nurse on 4-East tells me he's been asking for shots every hour, even though he knows the order restricts the injections to every three hours (I wrote q 3 h prn, grateful to have a vestigial remnant of our elite jargon). Examination is unchanged. He is still groaning and wincing continually. Liver tests are normal, white count is okay. The amylase level, a chemical probe for pancreatitis, is within normal limits.

"Dan, we're going to start with a couple of gallbladder tests. If the ultrasound shows no stones, we'll do a DESIDA scan to see if the gallbladder is blocked off.

"Anything, Doc, but can't I have something stronger for pain?" Now it's Doc.

"We'll see what we can do."

"Doc, my mother is coming from Little Rock, and she's bringing the reports and X-rays."

"Good -- is she flying in?"

"No -- driving. She should be here tomorrow."

"What's the name of the doctor who took care of you there?"

"Let's see. Madison. Lewis Madison."

Back in the office, with the telephone stack growing and with three patients already here for their appointments, I accost Sandra.

"Tell the telephone brigade I'll get to them later and explain to our guests that I'm running late. See if you can get a Dr. Lewis Madison in Little Rock on the phone. Tell his secretary it's about a patient named Dan Godwick."

"Wilco on number three. But of course numbers one and two have already been accomplished, dear doctor."

"Thank you, Sandra."   And thank you again, migraine.

AS HER WORLD TURNS

172

It's Natalie at the threshold. "They want orders on Karen. 415, you know."

"I know, I know. I'll call them over. The fax or computer never seem to deliver."

This is, of course, only one of many hospital admissions for Karen. After establishing herself in the legal world, she married a nice enough young fellow named Chris and two years later showed up pregnant. Simple enough, right? Wrong. One of the things guaranteed to strike terror into the hearts of an internist, nephrologist, rheumatologist or obstetrician is a lupus patient who gets pregnant. Why? one might ask -- doesn't the lupus actually get better during early pregnancy? Often. But it's the last three months, the last "trimester," that brings the incubus into her physicians' nights. For that's when the renal disease can flare, when the patient can get "toxemia." This means albumin in the urine, high blood pressure, generalized swelling, and sometimes kidney failure and convulsions. The blood pressure can be hard to treat -- you don't want to hurt the fetus with potent drugs. And for the same reason you hate to treat the lupus flare with high-doses of cortisone derivatives.

The only sure way out is early delivery; and very often the baby isn't ready yet. I remember coming to see Karen on the day of her admission to the OB unit. She was now 30. Her abdomen was appropriately big but her legs were swollen, (we say "4+ edema,") her blood pressure was 160/110. Her creatinine and BUN -- indices of kidney function -- were climbing out of range.

Full-term pregnancy is 38 weeks. Termination is usually safe beyond 32. Below that it's iffy.

Karen was 29 weeks along.

"I guess it's me or the baby, huh, Dr. Galen?"

"Come on, Karen, you've been watching *As the World Turns* or something.   We're working on you *and* the baby. You're going to lie around here until the OB doctors think little Mr. Chris, Jr., is OK for the light of day and then they'll bring him along one way or the other. They did tell you it's a he, didn't they?"

"Yes. The sonogram and all. But they said he's small. They want to wait until 32 weeks if they can. That's three weeks from now!"

"Don't worry, you can get the judge to continue your court cases."

"You always make me feel better, Dr. Galen."

"Dr. Feelgood, huh?"

"And a little more than that."

They did wait, Karen stayed in bed, and we kept her blood pressure in a respectable 140/90 range. But in ten days, not three weeks, nature moved in and brisk spontaneous labor came on. The OB people were pale. The pediatrician was even paler than usual (they seem to stay indoors a lot).

I went to the delivery room. It was the middle of the afternoon. As I walked in, I heard a vigorous high-pitched cry. "Chris, Jr.," was here.

And mother and son were fine.

For the moment.

To be sure, the kidney abnormalities cleared within three weeks. But four weeks postpartum Karen called and said she had to talk to me. Once in the office, she made a strange revelation.

"I haven't been able to tell anybody else this, Dr. Galen. Not mother, the OB group, anybody. But I know I'd better tell somebody, so I guess it has to be you. You're always the one who gets the bad news."

"Tell me, Karen."

"Well, I haven't been able to sleep. I have to force myself to eat. I've lost 15 pounds since I got out of the hospital."

"Do you feel --"

"There's something else a lot worse, Dr. Galen. I -- don't know how to say it."

"Just say it, Karen."

"All the time, all the time -- I find myself --"

"Yes?"

"Wanting to kill my baby!"

We arranged the best available treatment for her postpartum depression -- some call it psychosis, a strange and undoubtedly biochemically determined malady -- which ended up including a month of hospitalization and a longer period of separation from the child. Gradually, Karen was weaned back to motherhood and back to work. It was about eight months before she seemed completely recovered.

Her husband, Chris, Sr., never recovered. Maybe it was the lupus, the crisis, the bizarre reaction to his child, but in less than two years, they were divorced. Now Karen had the child and her job and the lupus. But somehow, she handled them all. She kept making the local papers from time to time with big cases. The little boy seemed to flourish.

At least in my office she never lost her bright smile. "We're going to make it, Dr. Galen. Will you still stick with us?"

"All the way, Karen. It's too late to get rid of me now."

FOUR ON THE FLOOR

There in the doorway Donna looks different: she is pale and her usual deference has been replaced by authoritative urgency. Or maybe terror.

"Dr. Galen, Dr. Williams needs you *now* in Room 3."

I dash around the corner, open the door of the examining room, and conclude that she is dead right. Rufus Conway, who moments ago said hello and shook my hand in the hallway, is sprawled on his back with Dr. Elbert Williams bent over him. Most impressive is Rufus' color. Normally almost as florid as red brick, he is now the hue of the mortar between them.

Dr. Elbert Williams' color is not too good either. "He's been having some left abdominal and flank pain, John. Exam of his abdomen was negative two minutes ago. Then he had sudden excruciating pain and he has no blood pressure."

We reexamine his belly. It is now quite tense, especially on the left. His left inguinal canal is bulging.

"Almost like an acute hernia," says Elbert.

176

We look at each other and we chant it together in a chorus:

"Ruptured aneurysm."

Then I put in, "But he's only, what, 52? Not hypertensive?"

"Fifty-four. And not hypertensive."

"Blood pressure 70 systolic now," says Donna.

"IV?" I say.

"Let's just get him to the ER first." The ER is only 200 feet away.

Sandra, on instruction, has already put in calls to the emergency room, to the general surgeon, Dr. Frank Wharton, and the vascular surgeon, Dr. Jardin. Wharton is the first to arrive.

From his position kneeling beside Rufus, Wharton looks at Williams and then at me. Surgeons may waste gauze sponges and disposable hemostats but they don't waste words.

"Aorta," he says.

The process of transferring Rufus turns out to be more complicated than it sounded. The doorway is narrow. Rufus weighs about 200. Williams is about 6'6". Wharton weighs about 230. I can see my role in this right off: I get out of the way.

Wharton and Williams rush Rufus by stretcher to the ER and I stay and man the fort. Dr. Boy is already in the hospital. They will start D-5-Ringers Lactate in two veins, call the vascular surgeon, get Rufus' blood pressure up, draw blood for type and cross-match, call the vascular surgeon again, accompany Rufus to the CT room for an emergency

177

abdominal scan, and notify the operating room they have one on the way. And call the vascular surgeon again.

As he pushes one end of the stretcher through the examining room, Williams, though wide-eyed and a little flushed, hasn't lost his perspective. He looks down at his patient and says:

"Rufus, we're not on automatic today."

"That right?" Rufus still looks like putty.

"Yeah. This is four on the floor."

NON-CONNECTION

" . . . Oh, Dr. Galen, information can't find a Dr. Lewis Madison in Little Rock, Arkansas," says Sandra, notepad in hand.

"Okay, maybe I've got it wrong. I'll check with Dan."

NO PERIODS

Reba comes in for a report on her recent physical. She will have a lot of questions, not because she has a lot of symptoms, but because of something unusual that happened in her life, something she has never gotten over.

When I first saw Reba, she was about 29 and was deeply disturbed about her physical condition. She had stopped having menstrual periods for eight years and had been unable to become pregnant. She had, of course, seen a number of doctors and was even then under hormonal therapy by a well-known endocrinologist in another city. On physical examination the only things that seemed amiss were

178

an increased amount of facial and body hair and a slightly enlarged clitoris.

I remember being discouraged: many women have borderline syndromes which include hirsutism (increased hair) and infertility; in most, treatment is frustrating. Nonetheless, without much enthusiasm I ordered tests of adrenal and ovarian function, just to be sure we weren't missing something big.

There was something big, all right. At that time, about the most sophisticated studies in this type of disorder were 24-hour urine values for hormone breakdown products (now you can order blood levels we didn't have then). Reba's were normal for 17-hydroxysteroids, but the 17-ketosteroids were phenomenal. With a normal range of about 4-12 mgm per 24 hours for women, Reba's was 141! This meant that somewhere, almost certainly, there was a tumor manufacturing huge quantities of male-type hormones, or androgens. No wonder she had no periods, was infertile, had too much body hair. No wonder she was frustrated and depressed: her body had been fighting off maleness for eight years.

Now the problem was to find the tumor. The two most likely spots by far were the ovary and the adrenal gland. Reba was thin and easy to examine, so both ovaries could be identified and felt to be normal in size. A sonogram would have been helpful here -- but it hadn't been invented yet. The adrenal glands, two little triangular hunks of tissue about the size of a chicken spleen, were a different story. Located above both kidneys, behind the abdominal viscera, covered

179

by the big back muscles, they are not available to the palpating hand. Today visualization of the adrenal glands, or of an adrenal tumor, is a snap: you order a CT scan or an MRI and get a beautiful anatomical display in twenty to sixty minutes. But back in 1966, such technology had never entered the dreams of the most visionary bioengineer. We had to go with an aortagram, in which contrast material is injected into the main vessel, the aorta, and the ramifications traced out. We did the test and there it was: a nice, Georgia-peach-sized mass above the right adrenal.

The rest was high drama. Gerald Pound, the surgeon, moved in. "We can get that out with no trouble," he pontificated. "I hope it's benign."

"Hope?" said Reba to me later. "In other words, it could be malignant?"

"Less than 20% chance of malignancy," I said. "The way it's behaved, I've got my money on an innocent tumor."

"I guess I've got more than just money on it," said Reba.

It was benign. Huge but benign. I went into Reba's room afterward with the surgeon to hear him describe the procedure. Now there are two ways surgeons describe a procedure they have just done: hard and easy. There's no in-between. The hard ones are usually painted in lurid colors: "Toughest case I've seen. Had to dissect for hours. Lot of bleeding. Difficult to find the tumor. Even then it had a complicated blood supply. Patient wasn't too stable throughout the procedure, blood pressure up and down. Had to give her six units. She's doing OK, though." Implicit in this dissertation, of course, is the subtle suggestion that the patient was lucky to have such an outstanding surgeon, that an ordinary operator would probably have been simply unable to carry it off.

But Reba's case, it seemed, was in the easy category. "No problem. Just shelled it out. Smooth as silk," said Gerald (*no problem for me*, he meant; *I made it look like a corn-shucking party; I am the one who's smooth*).

The denouement, of course, was happy (doctors like to tell you about their successes). Reba started having periods (and ovulating again). Then, the crowning achievement: she had a baby quite uneventfully.

And she named it after me! Me, who had more or less blundered into ordering a test. Naturally I went to the *briss,* which with all the goodies and the champagne and other wine essentially eliminated an ordinary weekday. As the cantor (with great skill) did the honors of the circumcision in the dining room, Reba's father came up close to me.

"You can see that we Jews are great optimists, Doctor."

"How's that, Mr. Kaplan?"

"Just look: we cut it off before we know how long it's going to be."

Now I'm able to tell Reba that all her studies, at 18 years' distance, are normal. Normal hormone tests. No masses.

"Congratulations, Reba. These days you're just a routine patient."

Reba is brunette, with bangs, wearing a blue suit with a red striped floppy tie. Just right for her job as account executive for the city's second-largest advertising agency. "Routine is what I've always hoped for, John. I don't like to be interesting in this office. By the way, you know that namesake of yours?"

"I sure do, Reba.

"He's going to Williams College."

"Great."

"The best part is, he's got an academic scholarship."

"Terrific."

"And you might be interested -- he thinks he wants to be a doctor."

"Yes, Reba. I am interested. Very. Thanks. And congratulations."

Reba jumps up, comments on the trailing plant in the corner, walks out my office door and into Irene's office. She is opening her pocketbook and taking out her checkbook.

You see, the incredible part is -- I'm actually going to get paid for this.

NO ANSWERS

There is still no progress on Dan Godwick except for the findings of a normal gallbladder ultrasound and DESIDA scan. He is just as frowny and wincy, just as uncomfortable.

"We'll have to do another retrograde and, if that's negative, an abdominal CT scan and an upper GI, Dan."

"I'm game, Doc, if you can just get me some relief."

I advance the Demerol to the sister drug Dilaudid, which some evidence indicates is more potent, put in a call to Walter Suttles, urologist, and move on.

LIABILITY AGAIN

The malpractice wraith surfaces in my mind, so I try Tom Whisenant again. In the ER parking lot, where no one will hear. Or so I hope.

"Woolrich, Heineman, Butler, and Whisenant, LLP," says the dulcet tone. LLP means Limited Liability Parnership. But they aren't really partners, I know. They don't trust anybody. What they have is a partnership of private corporations. They are doubly indemnified. You'd have to go through at least two layers of judicial insulation to get at any of those lawyers.

I dodge a car with a frantic-looking man at the wheel. "Mr. Whisenant back yet?"

"No, the court's running late, but I gave him your message. He was already trying to call you this morning."

Another car cruises by, just missing my left leg. "Yes, I know." I want to ask about what, but that would be sticking my toe in the inferno.

"Well, thanks. I'll wait for his call. Do you think it will be this evening?" An ambulance turns on its siren.

"Probably so," says dulcet.

This sets me to wondering what time cocktail hour is at WHB&W. Maybe I will get squeezed in. I close down the cell phone and make sure the charge is up.

VERY INTENSIVE CARE

Jimmy Treadway is deeply embedded in Unit 6 of the Med-Surg ICU, where he is surrounded by six health professionals doing a good imitation of that molecular dance known as Brownian motion. There are stalagmites and stalactites of IV poles arising from the floor and hanging from the ceiling. There is a ventilator, a portable X-ray juggernaut, and in the corner, a modern compact artificial kidney machine.

Eileen, the renal technologist, spies me and advances with her clipboard. "Want to give me some numbers, Dr. Galen, or shall I wing it?"

"Both, Eileen. I give you some numbers, then you wing it, and then I sign it, just like always. Seriously, we need a 2 K bath to start, then go to 3 after 2 hours if his level comes down under 5. No fluid removal right now – blood pressure's too shaky. Do you have a pretty big kidney – let's see, a K-300? That ought to work. Then the usual rules. I'll fill in the blanks." I take her clipboard.

"What kind of dialysis schedule do you expect from here on in?" Eileen asks.

"Every day for a week at least. Maybe more if the K gets out of hand. Even so we may not keep up with the various poisons. He needs a full-court press."

"Sure." She looks around the crowded cubicle. "So far, it looks like that's what he's getting."

BUT FIRST, DOCTOR

"Where is Mrs. Dan ---"

"But even before you see Mrs. Dandridge" -- Natalie likes to complete my sentences -- "Dr. Rhine is on 67."

"About --?"

"About Karen."

I pick the designer-beige instrument off the wall. I liked the old black ones. "Dan, what's new?"

Dan's answer provokes nostalgia about communications too -- it is reminiscent of the old Western Union telegram: "Got it open. Big clot. Slid right out with the Fogarty. Think she should be on heparin overnight. OK to go ahead and use it right away for dialysis."

"Terrific. She tolerate it OK?"

"Fine. No pain. Just used local."

"Great. But I mean, her emotional state holding up?"

"Guess so, I don't know, what am I, a psychiatrist?"

I start to say something really cross, then consider, No. I guess the psychiatrist is going to be me, but end up saying only,

"No, you aren't. You sure aren't. Thanks for everything."

Karen's psychiatric status, I recall, actually held up very well indeed after her episode of postpartum depression, and she only popped in for routine follow-up visits until, at ten a. m. one Tuesday morning four years ago, I got a call.

"Dr. Galen, I'm getting paralyzed."

It's not unusual for patients to complain of paralysis, when what's really happening is something else: bursitis in the shoulder makes the arm too painful to move; swelling of

185

the leg makes it seem immobile, etc. But Karen is different --
first, she's all too experienced with illness, and, second, she
has an IQ off the top of the Stanford-Binet scale.

"Where, Karen?"

"Well, first, my feet were clumsy, then my knees,
then my thighs, then my lower lumbar muscles. Now I'm
having trouble breathing."

Dear God.

On top of everything else, Guillain-Barre syndrome!

"Get someone to bring you to the hospital, Karen. Go
to the Emergency Room. Bring your toothbrush, we'll
probably keep you a while."

"I figured. I'm already packed."

By the time we saw Karen she was mildly to
moderately weak in all her muscles except those of the neck
and face -- it hadn't gotten up there yet. Her breathing, though
adequate, was definitely shallow as revealed by the portable
spirometer. It could get shallower, we knew -- even stop
entirely -- so she was placed in the ICU on a respiratory
monitor and ear oximetry. Thus her breathing pattern was
reflected on a screen and an alarm went off if it
dropped
below a critical level. A little clamp with a light in it was
clipped like an earring to her right earlobe, leading to a very
clever electronic monitor which read out her oxygen
saturation, second by second, on a big digital display: 90%,
92%, 91%, 95%, etc. You don't want it to drop, and stay,
below 90%.

186

If she wasn't moving the right amount of air we wanted to know it. Right away. Then we'd have to support her -- put an endotracheal tube down her windpipe, blow up a little balloon to make it tight, hook it up to a ventilator, breathe for her until she recovered.

Indeed, the neurologist Walter Armstrong and I agreed: the clinical picture was certainly identical to the syndrome described by the French physicians Guillain and Barre' -- a pattern of rapidly advancing ascending paralysis. Though the cause is strictly speaking unknown, it is generally agreed that a virus starts it off, probably by triggering an immune reaction of the body against its own nervous system. The picture may be mild, as was the case so far with Karen, or it may result in complete immobilization of every muscle in the body. Recovery occurs in about 80 percent of patients, but it may take days or weeks; the other 20 percent have a variable outcome – from weakness here and there up to quadriplegia.

The other characteristic of this bizarre disease is found in the cerebrospinal fluid. If you do a spinal tap you find a great increase in the amount of protein there; instead of about 20 mgm per 100 ml, it may be 300. In most other conditions this only happens when there is a big collection of inflammatory cells in the fluid, as in meningitis; in Guillain-Barre, there are no cells, only the high protein. This curious finding is of great value to the neurologist because, among other things, it permits him to unleash one of his most cherished of all terms: "albumino-cytologic dissociation of the spinal fluid." I think they spend a prescribed amount of time during training teaching and practicing the articulation of this phrase; they have to say it just right or they don't get their certificates.   It's just as essential to the neurologist as the carefully cultivated "Gawd" is to the minister or "twit" (for *to wit*) is to the lawyer.

Walter went ahead with the spinal tap on Karen and then he called me with the results.

"She had only two cells, John, but her protein was 312 mgm%."

I waited expectantly for the hallowed phrase.

But Walter was too sophisticated, or thought I was. "Typical of the G-B syndrome."

"Right. But you know, all her lupus indices are up -- high sed rate, ANA, anti-DNA, complement. Could this be coming from lupus rather than the usual virus or whatever?"

Always thinking, you see.

"Possible." But Walter was ready for me. "I've already done a Medline library search. There've been three cases like this in the world literature in the last ten years -- the Guillain-Barre syndrome due to lupus."   Phrases weren't all Walter learned in training.

We treated her with "pulse" steroids -- high-dose, intravenous infusions -- and she cleared completely within five days. No respirator. No permanent effects. (Nowadays we'd do plasmapheresis – remove the plasma from the blood and replace it with an innocent saline-albumin solution, but that wasn't in vogue then.)

188

"We did it again, Dr. Galen," she said through her typical brilliant smile after transfer to a private room.

"Yep. But this time you warned me."

"You mean by calling you?"

"No, I mean some time back, after your psycho spell."

'What did I say?"

"You said you might have another weird episode."

TESTS NEGATIVE

Once again I stand at Dan Godwin's bedside. The retrograde was normal -- no stones, no anything. The abdominal CT scan was negative -- no abscess, no renal carbuncle. Upper GI series was clear -- no ulcer. He still has no fever and repeat blood tests remain normal.

But Dan is still writhing.

"Just can't get over this pain. Can't sleep a wink."

"You're getting the maximum doses of pain relievers, Dan. Maybe we can give you a sedative in addition. So far we can't find anything. When do you expect your mother?"

"Oh, I meant to tell you, her car broke down in Alabama, Doc. Maybe she can get here tomorrow or the next day."

"Okay. By the way, we can't find a Dr. Lewis Madison in Little Rock."

"Oh, that's right. He came in from Fort Smith. That's where he has his office, I think."

DYSINFORMATION

Mr. Rackley has been sent straight to my office because I'm running late. When I walk in to give the report on his physical examination, he moves around briskly, looks at his watch. He seems to have the idea his time is worth more than mine. Since he is the personnel director of a large accounting firm, with about 950 bodies to manage, he's undoubtedly right.

"Sorry I'm late. You probably wouldn't put up with that from any of your subordinates, would you?"

"You'd be amazed what I put up with, Dr. Galen, but everybody knows about doctors. You're not as bad as most. I have plenty of work here." He motions to his briefcase. "Brought it on purpose."

"Good. Well, down to business, your physical exam was quite good. Blood pressure up a little -- we'll come back to that. Heart, lungs, abdomen -- all fine. Proctoscopic exam showed nothing significant. Complete blood count OK -- no anemia. Blood chemistries normal across the board: no diabetes, liver function OK, kidneys fine, electrolytes within normal limits. Cholesterol is in a good range." Here I expect an interruption, and I get one.

"What *was* my cholesterol, Doctor, and my tri-glyceride level?" Everybody knows about cholesterol, or thinks he does. It's considered the be-all and the end-all as far as health is concerned.

"Your cholesterol is 208 milligrams per 100 milliters. Normal is 150 to 240, but we like it below 200 if possible. Yours is satisfactory, could be a little lower. The LDL (bad cholesterol) is the main thing we worry about these days, and yours is 98 – very good. Anything below 130 is acceptable."

"Well, but Pritikin says my total cholesterol should be 100 plus my age, and I'm only 42. How do I get it down to 142? And also they say your LDL should be way below 100."

Sometimes I think I'll log in all the minutes I spend trying to disabuse people of the rich storehouse of misinformation they have acquired with the marvelously inventive assistance of the press and internet. Just the time I took to write it down would probably put me out of business.

"Well, sir, first of all, the only people who go around with a cholesterol under 150 are in one of the following categories: one, rural Chinese subsisting off a rice-and-fish diet; two, people who are starving as a result of cancer, or some type of intestinal or liver disease which prevents them from utilizing their foodstuffs; three, war prisoners who really are starving; four, people who have happened to inherit the tendency for such a low value from their parents; and, finally, five, people on a freak diet like that designed by the Pritikin people. By the way, based on my experience with patients who have gone into that program full blast, that born-again philosophy only lasts a few months until they go back to a more typical American program.

"You also ought to know that a lot of people with a cholesterol of 290 live to be 90, and I had a man with a cholesterol of 155 admitted to the hospital with a massive heart attack last week. Needed a quadruple bypass."

"Really?"

"Yes. But that's just to point out that the level of cholesterol in the bloodstream is just one factor. You've got to figure on the high and low-density lipoproteins. On this score, you look good."

"Great."

"But more important are all the other factors. The two most important are one you can't help and one you can."

"What's that?"

"Your family history of heart attack and stroke. You can't alter that, can't pick your ancestors. But fortunately, you seem to have done pretty well in the game of genetic roulette."

"Yes, no big problems in the family that I know of."

"And the smoking of cigarettes."

"Yes, I know that. Guess everybody does. I smoke about a pack a day. Is that too much?"

"Any is too much. Smoking is the number one reversible factor underlying heart attack, strokes, and other forms of atherosclerosis."

"Really?"

"Really. When they studied the coronary angiograms -- that is, pictures of heart arteries -- right after, and two years after, heart bypass surgery, the films fell out into two groups: those that stayed the same and those that got worse over the study period."

"Just two years?"

"Just two years. They studied every factor known to influence these changes, from heredity to triglycerides to caffeine to stress."

"And?"

"And only one factor seemed to be critical."

"What was it?"

"The worsening group was those who kept smoking and the stable group was those who didn't."

"How am I going to quit, Doctor? They have all kinds of programs."

"True. And I'd encourage you to try any you think might help, including certain drugs we have now. But there's only one thing that's going to do it."

"What?"

"Re-identify yourself as a non-smoker. Win the war. Don't fight fifty battles a day -- sooner or later you'll lose."

"I'll start on it--soon. But you said something about my blood pressure."

I move to his side and recheck the blood pressure with my sphygmomanometer. "Yes, it's a little high--145 over 98. The other day it was 150 over 100. Previously it's been normal -- in the 110 to 120 over 76 to 86 range. We'll need to get a longer-term blood pressure record to find out what your average levels really are, in your normal life pattern. Nowadays, studies show we want it to be in the 120/80 range if at all possible. If it's up, we may need to check out some tests to be sure why, especially at your age and since you have no family history."

"At my age? You mean because I'm so young?"

"No, nothing personal, but because you're so old."

"What do you mean by that?"

I laugh a little. "You see, most so-called essential, or inherited, hypertension shows up earlier than this, maybe even to some extent in teen-age. At your age we have to think about kidney artery trouble, or a tumor of the adrenal gland, things like that. We certainly don't to want a miss a curable form of high blood pressure before we start treating it."

"Yes, well, I agree. I certainly, above all, don't want to start on any blood pressure medicines."

"You don't?"

"Certainly not. I would want the alternative method of bringing blood pressure down. I just read a book about it."

Here we go again. "Did that book suggest that exercise, and weight control, and the relief of unnecessary stress, and avoiding salt was the alternative pathway to blood pressure control?"

"Well, yes, that was essentially it."

"Then I must tell you two things about that. First, it is not an alternative way. It's the standard way. We always employ those basic principles before considering drug therapy."

"Oh. I'm relieved to hear that."

"And the second thing is that these methods alone only work in about ten per cent of cases of true hypertension."

"That's not what this book said."

"No, it wouldn't. After all, the author's primary goal was to sell books."

"Why, they wouldn't let someone publish a book like that unless it were true, would they?"

"Who's *they,* Mr. Rackley? Most of the vast literature which appears on the streets every day is either partially false, quite misleading, or sufficiently flawed as to convey more incorrect than true information. There are 100,000 websites on the internet for health and 95% have no credentials – they're written by Ben the grocer or whoever. The reasons for this are hard to figure out. Maybe it's because the writers and editors are more concerned about readership than leadership. And then I have another hypothesis."

"What's, that, Dr. Galen?"

"That most of the people who go into journalism did so because they didn't like biology. And the science writers -- there's something special about them."

"What?"

"I think they are chosen from the flunkees."

But what I don't tell Mr. Rackley is that many people continue to believe what they read even after the doctor tells them otherwise. Maybe it's the power of the written word. Strange, since every survey indicates doctors are high, and journalists are low, on the "trust" list. Maybe it's the physician's failure to inject that essential element of fantasy. He sticks to dusty, unimaginative, usually unappealing realities. He tells you that calories *do* count. Ugh! That "light" cigarettes are still bad for you. That "light" beer is just low-alcohol beer (near-beer). That aspirin is aspirin, no matter how advertised, decorated, or ballyhooed. That the 30-pound weight gain is not fluid. That there is no simple blood test for cancer. The doctor has the medieval idea that a negative prostatic ultrasound does not insure against cancer of that organ, and even harbors the disgustingly pedestrian notion that the palpating finger is probably better (and much cheaper). He even knows that the PSA test may lie – about 15% of the time. Primitive that he is, the physician may not think a CT scan will help a migraine-sufferer. He has the temerity to suggest that a cardiac PET scan, which made the front page when a local hospital got one, is not the touchstone for heart disease; indeed he has the arrogant skepticism to tell the patient that it has not yet been proved to add much.

I arrange for Mr. Rackley to get serial blood pressure determinations and to enroll in a local quit-smoking program. I urge him to get some regular aerobic exercise.

On the way out he turns and asks: "Oh, Doctor, can't I just get one of those shots to get me off cigarettes?"

"There really aren't any shots that work, Mr. R." Then I ask, knowing the answer: "Where did you hear about shots for stopping smoking?"

"I read about it on the internet, let's see . . . ."

ANOTHER CALL

It's Natalie again.

". . . and no Lewis Madison in Fort Smith. In fact, no Lewis Madison in the Arkansas Medical Society roster."

"Guess it's time to quit cutting bait and start fishing."

"I love your archaic metaphors, Dr. Galen."

"I'm a little busy right now, Natalie. Can we discuss my rhetoric later?"

"Sure. I'll be right there at my usual station."

DAILY DOLDRUMS

The creeping fatigue -- I doubt if it could be ennui -- announces four o'clock. I wonder why this is the nadir of my every day: the pencil suddenly a leaden sceptre, the stethoscope a silver-and-rubber albatross clinging about the strap muscles, the last patient a dreaded fardel. Just tired, you say? Why then the rejuvenation by 5:30? Psychic release, you explain -- you're through with your day, the prospect of home beckons. But I will not be through, not nearly; there is no release; there is no home for hours yet.

No, my friend, four p.m. is the neurohumoral snake pit of humankind: the plasma cortisol, pulsed to its zenith by the early-morning burst of pituitary corticotropin, has, alas, waned. The five-a.m. squirt of androgens -- fostered by a different trophic hormone, but from the same pituitary master gland -- has settled obsequiously into tissue receptor sites or been metabolized into impotent fragments. Surely there is an even more cogent circulating factor, as yet undiscovered, which provides verve, inspiration, intellectual initiative, secreted perhaps by a group of highly specialized nerve cells at the base of, let's say, the pineal gland in the midbrain (the pineal always gets credit for anything mysterious). These cells must fire off at five a.m., begin again at noon, and not until six p. m. do they ejaculate their final burden of revivifying substance into the blood stream. Certainly Vivaldi was riding high on some lovely peptide as *The Four Seasons* flowed from his scratchy quill; Hamlet, depressed

197

though he was, could never have instructed us on enterprises of great pith and moment had his creator not been tripping out on pinealamine or whatever. Wyeth? His watercolors would have surely run together like mud had he essayed even the simplest barn at quarter after four (unless, perchance, Helga had been perched on a nearby bale). And yet here I sit in my black leather desk chair -- limp, depleted, biochemically bereft, victim of my own hormonal rhythmicity.

But four o'clock Thursday afternoon is nonetheless infinitely superior to the same hour on Saturday or Sunday if one should be "on call." Then, cursed with the demon of being "in the barrel" for several doctors, one faces the challenge which I have come to call the "geriatric discovery phenomenon." This entity consists of a series of illnesses, disabilities, distresses, and annoyances which seem at this curious juncture to affect only the very old. They may have pneumonia, urinary infection, worsening of their heart failure, malnutrition, bad colds, dehydration, whatever. And you may already be framing in your mind your perceptive question: How could these morbid processes, all typically gradual, suddenly reach the critical moment of hospital admission or a trip to the emergency clinic at a single stroke of the hour hand? That low cortisone level? Hardly. Four p. m. on a weekend day is the time when you go see granny, or your aging aunt, and find out how bad she's been for a week or two. But, you see, action at teatime Saturday still allows you to get to the party. Sunday afternoon, on the other hand, adds a new dimension: get things squared away so you won't miss work Monday: "Doctor, it's clear grandpa just needs to be in

198

the hospital." (Translation: "*I* need for him to be in the hospital.")

The terrors of the weekend are by no means limited to this gerontological onslaught, however. These two days will bring people outdoors, where they can easily inflict upon themselves countless unexpected injuries; where the aging athlete can discover the lost resilience in his Achilles tendons. But the weekend has its own special psychic wonders, too: it galvanizes the insane streak in every patient. One Saturday was so impossible recently that I had to write up a bulletin for one of our associates whose patients, it proved, were the prime offenders. It was fatuously designed to be posted in his reception room wall. The text appears below:

NOTICE
ATTENTION: ALL POTENTIAL PATIENTS
OF DR. LANDERS

Welcome!

However, if you are applying to become a regular patient, you should be aware of the strict criteria you must meet. You must agree to conform to a minimum of four (4) of the following six (6) stipulations:

*1.	You should call him frequently but must avoid calling him during regular business hours when at all possible. And while it is technically permissible to call Dr. Landers himself at night and on weekends, it is far preferable to call when he is off call and speak to one of his associates who has never heard of you. With a little experience, you may be able to join the raft of people who, at 5:10 p.m. on Friday, call to have their regular prescriptions renewed by 5:30. It is, of course, not essential to call at that specific hour; instead, 1 a. m. Sunday morning or 5 a. m. on Saturday morning are equally acceptable alternatives.*

199

2. If you have a problem which has become chronic, you may be tempted to call Dr. Landers' office, make a convenient appointment, and arrange to have him evaluate and treat the difficulty under optimal conditions. Do not yield to this temptation! It is imperative here to delay consultation as long as possible and then, on a weekend, insist on being seen by the alternative physician. Please note that calling on Dr. Landers' evening off may not be satisfactory: the physician may callously suggest that, since the problem is non-urgent, you wait and call your regular doctor in the morning. Observe that he cannot do this if you call at, say, suppertime on Friday night. Again, pre-dawn hours on Saturday will suffice.

An example of an eminently successful recent operation of this kind was Mr. BS, who called Dr. JG at 9 p.m. on Friday night, described a cold which had been present for two months, and insisted on being seen the next morning, saying he had seen Dr. Landers three times without success. Indeed, the next day in the emergency room, he did indeed (1) have a cold; he had indeed (2) seen Dr. Landers three times (but not this year); and (3) actually wanted a shot to prevent pneumonia. While it is recognized that not all physician-contact opportunities can be this wonderfully contrived, this is listed here as an ideal toward which to aspire.

3. Be careful, when receiving physical exam reports from Dr. Landers, to obtain only a fraction of your values. Wait until another doctor is on call and beep him on the pager. Then, as blandly as possible, request to know your blood sugar, cholesterol, and BUN. If you can do this without actually identifying yourself as other than "Jimmy" or "Fanny," your status will rise in this office. Additional points are awarded if you actually beep the doctor as an emergency.

4. This item is a variation on 3. If you have a condition likely to cause bizarre lab values -- such as diabetes and you ignore your diet, or if you have kidney failure and you skipped a dialysis -- try to come in for regular lab tests late Friday afternoon. In this way the regular run at Doctors' Lab will be completed at about 11 p.m. and critical lab values, like your sky-high blood sugar or your soaring potassium, will be phoned urgently to the doctor on call. This has several advantages. First, allowing for the answering service delay, the doctor will be beeped at about 11:45 p. m.; second, because it is announced as a critical value, the service may send it through as an emergency; and, third, since the physician never heard of you or your problem, he may feel compelled to call you and/or Dr. Landers. If you can arrange this at a time when both you and Dr. Landers are out of town, you may be eligible for a substantial discount on your bill.

5. Arrange to phone the on-call doctor from another city as often as possible. If you can leave the out-of-town number without the area code, this is worth extra points. Ideally, the occasion should be minor, such as hay fever, and you should request that the call be returned "As Soon As Possible" (abbreviated ASAP) so that you can get to the wedding. Never have the drug store number available. Tell the doctor it's the Acme Drug Store on Ocean Drive and doesn't he have a Sea Island directory? One of our recent legendary triumphs occurred when a lady called a new on-call physician at 6 a.m. on Sunday morning from Hilton Head, said she felt a little headachy, and did he think she should play tennis later on that day?

6. Special consideration is given to those patients who call multiple times about the same problem. For example, if, after developing a routine cold, you can call Friday night about the sniffles, Saturday morning about sinus congestion, Saturday night about the sore throat, Sunday morning about the post-nasal drip, and Sunday night about the cough, you will have accumulated bonus points. If you can arrange to carry out the foregoing sequence while Dr. Fitzgibbon is on call, you may even be excused from criteria 1-5. (Dr. Fitzgibbon is quite intolerant of such calls.)

Nobody is perfect, and we don't expect everyone to be able to accomplish all of the above all the time. But we want you to understand you are joining an elite corps of performers. Let's don't allow the quality to deteriorate.

201

Little David, it has to be admitted, fielded this hot grounder with a great deal of aplomb: he had it copied and handed it out to all his patients for an entire week. Most of the recipients laughed loudly.

Unfortunately, the most deserving patients didn't get one.

SURGERY CONSULT

I walk into the 4-East nursing station dreading the latest report on my problem-child Dan Godwin.

Frank Wharton, general surgeon, has seen Dan at my request. His note on the chart is characteristically succinct: "R abd. and flank pain 24 h. No guarding, no significant tenderness, normal bowel sounds, normal WBC, GB sonogram, DESIDA, UGI, CT abd scan. Impression: no surgical indication at present. Continue observation."

So that's it, eh, Frank -- no need to operate now, so therefore what? No surgical problem? What the hell is wrong, then? He's still hurting, writhing, getting narcotics.

Back at the bedside, I decide to exorcise, from the back of my brain, the wraith which has been growing and nagging there for 12 hours.

"Dan, are you ready to level with me yet?"

"What do you mean, Doctor?" Apparently I've been promoted from Doc.

"You know what I mean."

"No, all I know, I just have this pain."

"Okay, I'm cutting the pain medication now and gradually we'll taper it off. We don't find anything wrong."

"But I'm suffering."

"You'll suffer more if you stay on these drugs."

At the nursing station, I cut the Dilaudid from two to one milligram "q 3 h prn."

"For you, Dr. Galen." Nurse Cantwell hands me the abhorred black instrument. It is Jean Snare, head of patient accounts. Jean doesn't know much about abdominal pain or sonograms, but she knows all about insurance and people's ability to pay their hospital bills.

"This patient was in here two weeks ago, Dr. Galen. Dr. Houston had him in. Abdominal pain. Tests negative. Nurses recorded a lot of injections. Signed out against medical advice when Dr. Houston cut off the shots. Gave the name of Don Goodwin. Same birth date, though. Oh, and also, in checking on his insurance--"

"Yes?"

"They can't find him on the student list at State Tech. Thought you ought to know."

"Sure, Glenda. Thanks. Put the chart in my box, will you?"

HEROES AND OTHERS

"I guess we're finished with the patients, then, Sandra?" I push back from the desk. "Thank goodness."

"Well, Dr. Galen, the scheduled patients, yes, but you know you've got the conference with the Jakes family about the kidney transplant thing."

Jakes -- yes, Charles Jakes. He is an amazing guy. Blind since age 11 from congenital corneal disease, he nonetheless built a successful shop in which he sells musical instruments, including pianos. He also moves them, tunes them, plays them. He can perform competently on six other musical instruments, which he does for his own amusement. His firm employs about 40 people. Just to fill his spare time, he has an elaborate ham radio system. As if his ocular deficit weren't enough, nature cursed him with kidney disease which last year progressed to end-stage kidney failure. He has been on that form of the artificial kidney known as hemodialysis, three times a week, and he hates every second of it; consequently, the wonderful women in dialysis nursing who treat him hate it *for* him. So we've been talking about transplantation, whether from a relative or from a cadaver. He said "maybe one of" his siblings would volunteer to be tested.

"You mean the brother and sister or whoever to talk about giving a kidney?" I ask Sandra. "Well, send them back."

"Dr. Galen, you don't exactly understand. I can't just -- send them back." Sandra gets that faint smile and that faint blush. She's one of those who can still blush. I like that.

"Why not?"

"They're out in the waiting room, and --"

"And?"

204

"They fill it up. There are eleven brothers and sisters out there." The smile is broader now and the blush is deeper. "They'd never get in your office."

The whole group is sitting around the reception room, and everybody stands up when I come in.   Some people would call these folks "country."   I call them friendly, attentive, intelligent -- and something else. Charles is absent on my suggestion; I told him I wanted to "talk turkey." After I finish my fifteen-minute spiel on what it means to give up a kidney -- providing luxuriant details about possible (though unlikely) complications such as post-operative infection, clots to the lung, later damage to the remaining kidney, etc. -- I decide the adjective which best describes this crowd is *undismayed.*

"Better take mine, Doc," says a tall, lean man with straight, scanty hair. He pulls at his old-fashioned overalls. "I'm the black sheep."

There is loud laughter all around, the kind that comes only after long practice.

Another says, "He might just reject your kidney on general principles, Carey." More laughter.

"I do have one question, Doc," says a younger brother, who is still wearing his baseball-style Federated Warehouse cap.

"Sure, Mr. Jakes," I say.

"If I turn out to be the one, will my company insurance pay for any of this?"

I explain that not only should his insurance apply, but federal Medicare has a provision that will allow 100%

205

reimbursement for donor and recipient -- about the only condition where such a liberal federal policy exists.

"That's good, Doc," he goes on. "'Cause I just have this job on the loading dock. I don't make a whole lot, and I was just gonna say . . . ." He starts laughing again.

"Say what, Mr. Jakes?"

"That if they ain't gonna' pay, you might as well just go ahead and take out both kidneys while you're in there." Again, they laugh. This time I laugh, too. Funny how laughing sometimes causes your eyes to water.

The Jakes remind me of the fact that there is no situation which peels back the well-covers of human courage like the kidney transplant process. People with a lifelong pattern of ordinariness suddenly and with no ceremony whatever vault into a mythological level of heroism. While the reverse can also be true -- a young man desperately needs a donor and the whole family become unaccountably silent -- I continue to be amazed at the human resources which lie there unannounced.

Like the Ben Findley case. Young Ben's kidney, transplanted from his father, lasted nine years, then began to fail. Biopsy -- in which a small needle sample of the tissue is taken and studied under conventional and electron microscopy – showed not rejection reaction but recurrence of the original disease.

Ben's father caught my sleeve in the hall of the hospital. "Looks like he took my kidney pretty well, after all," said the big, burly farm-implement dealer. "I'm 66 years old, Doctor. Ben's 32. Why don't you just take my other kidney for him and let me go on dialysis?"

I don't know exactly what I said, maybe nothing. Maybe I couldn't say anything. Ben eventually got a cadaver graft and is doing well again. His dad, of course, still has his own remaining kidney.

And something more.

I think back some twenty-five years, to 1964, to the time before chronic dialysis and before kidney transplantation. The management of renal failure then was purely supportive: diet, medications, try to keep the kidneys going as long as possible, look for any reversible components, make the patient comfortable. Then -- uremia, or uremic poisoning, as the more dramatic would have it, would set in. And coma. And death. I think of the many patients whom I watched drift down this discouraging hill. And, at this moment, I think of Mr. Jasper.

On that afternoon in the intensive care unit of the medical center I looked at Mr. Jasper and I know the inevitable had happened. He had deep, stertorous respiration. He looked pale. He had whitish flakes over his face and neck, which had appeared since the previous night. His blood chemistries showed a blood urea nitrogen (BUN) of 178 mgm/dl. His breath had a sick metallic odor. I knew all these findings were part of the same thing: the flakes were urea crystals, deposited on the skin because the kidneys aren't excreting it; the BUN was up for the same reason; the breath odor was, again, urea. The deep respiration was from the acidosis that accompanies chronic kidney insufficiency.

I had known Mr. Jasper was headed this way for several years. He had appeared with albumin and red blood cells in his urine, and a kidney biopsy had showed a disease known as membranoproliferative glomerulonephritis, a disorder with an unknown cause and no cure. I had discussed it with him and his family, told them we'd fight it, do everything to keep the kidney function up as much as possible, but that progression was inevitable.

And here we were, with only days to spare before intoxication with his own waste products would lead Mr. Jasper to death. Sadly, I wrote orders for control of nausea, carefully calculated the IV fluids, and walked outside to talk with his wife and children.

Mrs. Jasper, the son, Jim, and the daughter, Allie, were there. They looked as resigned as I felt.

"Well, it looks like we're getting near the end," I said softly. "Of course, uremia is usually fairly kind. The patient lapses into a stupor, like a light sleep, and then very often the potassium goes up to high levels and the heart just stops. The only thing we could do now would be a temporizing measure. We could use the artificial kidney to remove the poisons from his system. We could even use it several times. But I'm afraid that would only prolong things for days, maybe a couple of weeks. I'm going to have to talk to him about it. After all, he'll have to make the decision."

"Oh, yes, Doctor Galen," said Mrs. Jasper. "You ask him. But I know he won't want that. Unless there's some chance for him to get better for months, or a year, or longer?"

"Not that I can see. But strange things happen sometimes. And of course we never want to get in the way of a miracle."

Just then a man walked up and joined the group. I turned to him, then stepped back aghast. It was *the patient*, Ray Jasper! I started to explain that he was too ill to get up and leave the unit by himself, that he was unsteady, could fall, when Mrs. Jasper put her hand on my arm.

"Dr. Galen, this is Ray's brother, Walter."

"I guess you'd say I did a double take, Mr. Jasper. Are you two -- identical twins?"

"That's what they say, Doctor."

"I never knew Ray had a twin -- a brother and sister, sure. But a twin." I felt my pulse accelerating and the blood rush to my face.

The family shifted around from foot to foot there in the waiting room of the intensive care unit. They seemed confused, they wondered what was wrong with me. "Mr. Jasper -- Walter -- could you come over to my office this afternoon? I'd like to -- uh -- fill you in on Ray's situation a little more."

"Sure, Doctor, sure." Walter looked as quizzical as the others.

Two hours later he appeared in my office, and there, with the door closed, I explained the amazing fact -- that, even at that primitive stage of development, successful kidney transplantation between identical twins was being performed in Boston. Was he willing to be considered as a donor? Of course. If not, no one will even know he refused. No, no, Doctor, I' d do anything for Ray. Was he healthy as far as he knew? Healthy as a horse, Doctor.

Then I checked his blood pressure: 110/76. I personally took his urine specimen into the lab. With a small prayer I added Robert's Reagent to check for protein, spun the urine in a centrifuge, and spread the sediment out on a slide to study under the microscope. For, marvelous as the coincidence of the twinship was, there remained the horrifying possibility -- even likelihood -- that the two men had the identical disease.

The protein was negative and the sediment was clear.

The rest, at least for me, would be easy. We would contact Peter Bent Brigham Hospital in Boston. We would have chromosomal matching done to prove the fact that Walter and Ray were homozygotic -- in other words, came from the same egg (nowadays DNA mapping would be even more secure). We'd study Walter's health status, X-ray his kidneys, make sure he understood the risks of organ donation, and send him to Boston for final clearance. If, as seemed likely, he passed the rigorous tests, a transplant could be done within weeks.

Meanwhile, that day, we did indeed start dialyzing Ray on the artificial kidney. We would keep him in reasonable health until time to go to Boston. As I had told the family, strange things happen sometimes.

And you never want to get in the way of a miracle.

And then there was Mrs. Hauman. At 72 years of age, she had to hear from me that her rectal bleeding was due to malignancy. She'd have to have major surgery, then probably radiation, and then the inevitable silence that follows all assaults on cancer . . . the terrible, endless wait for the crucial but not-so-magic five years. First she had to go see her brother in Maine, she said, then she'd come back for the operation.

Weeks later, when I arrived on the nursing unit where Mrs. Hauman had just been admitted, the nurse walked up and in a low voice asked, "Did you hear about Mrs. Hauman's brother?"

I said I hadn't.

"He had colon cancer. She went to nurse him. He just died."

I walked into the room. "Mrs. Hauman, I'm so sorry about your brother. And I'm particularly sorry you had to go through all that just before your own operation."

"That's all right, doctor. It's worked out fine."

"How do you mean?"

"I mean, watching him suffer through all that and trying to help and everything."

"Yes?"

"It's given me strength to deal with my own problem."

I think the ultimate reward was Joyce. She was now in her forties, blind, brilliant, and on dialysis on the artificial kidney. She was also the most buoyant soul around; she

211

could cheer up the most depressed fellow-patient, the most harried nurse, or the most stressed-out doctor.

One day I heard her family home had burned down. I sat down and took her hand.

"Joyce, what can I say? I'm so sorry. At least nobody was hurt."

"Yes, Doctor Galen, and this has helped me to understand my blindness. . .in three ways."

"How, Joyce?"

"Well, mother and Dad couldn't see to dial the phone, but I didn't need to see."

"Because you could dial 911 without seeing."

"Right. And they couldn't see to get out of the house, so I just led them."

"Because you could find your way without seeing. Wonderful, Joyce. But you said three things?"

"Yes. We sat outside in the yard."

"Yes?"

"And I didn't even have to see the house burn down."

I walked back out to the nursing station and turned to my own problems. The only thing was, I just couldn't seem to think of any.

KAREN FLARES

Natalie has a stack of charts in her arms as she stands in front of my desk but her faraway look tells me she's not thinking about any of them.

"Boy trouble? Or planning your vacation?"

"Sir?" She looks wide-eyed.

212

"You seem to be gathering moss."

"Oh, no." She laughs, briefly.

"I was thinking about Karen still."

"Don't blame you."

"How did her kidneys fail? Wasn't she in pretty good shape about, oh, a year ago? She seemed OK when she'd come in here."

"Yes. Did real well for the most part for about 25 years. Then it happened."

"It?"

"The full-blown lupus flare. Crash, you might call it. Called up one day, said she had fever, hurting all over. Like the flu. But it wasn't the flu."

"It was lupus cutting loose." Natalie sits down in one of the orange leather chairs.

"Right. Got her in here. BP sky-high. Fever. Joints inflamed. Butterfly on her face, red rash all over her torso. Anemia. Low white count. Albumin in the urine. Creatinine and BUN shooting up. Put her in the hospital, started her on high-dose cortisone derivatives. Did a kidney biopsy. Gave her 'pulse' steroids."

"Did she get better?"

"Generally, yes. Her kidneys, no. Biopsy showed the bad kind of lupus nephritis, what we call proliferative nephritis. And also vasculitis -- inflammation of the blood vessels. This meant arteries all over the body were involved."

"Could you treat that?"

"To some extent. We gave her cyclophosphamide. It's a toxic drug but sometimes it works like a charm."

213

"Did it?"

"With everything but the kidneys. They went downhill and eventually shut down completely. And here we are."

"How did she take to dialysis?"

"Poorly. She adopted a positive attitude -- you know how she is -- said she'd dialyze as long as necessary, then go for a kidney transplant. But she got severely depressed again, started back with a psychiatrist. She's a 110-per-cent performer and anything which gets in her way, like three-time-a-week stints on the machine for three hours gets her down."

"I could see that."

LIABILITY STILL

The cell phone tinkles.

"Galen here."

"John, Tom Whisenant."

"Hi, Tom." Something moves in the pit of my stomach again. " What's up?".

"A lot. You remember this Caisson case?

Remember? My hands are sweating. "Sure."

"He filed a Chapter 11."

"Oh, really? Probably will allege that I'm the reason he had to go bankrupt."

"He probably would. They wanted to put the case off longer."

"Hell, it's been two and a half years and his lawyer hasn't even bothered to arrange a time to take my deposition." Now my armpits are sweating.

"Right. I pointed this out and moved for a dismissal."

"You did? What did the judge, uh, court, rule?"

"He dismissed it."

"Really? Does that mean I'm off the hook on this?"

"Yep."

"Great."

"With one small caveat."

"What's that?"

"He can refile within six months."

"And start the whole thing over?"

"And start the whole thing over."

"Do you think he will?"

"Probably not. But we never know, John. We never know."

EVIL EYE

As I dry my brow, I remember the time when the hospital risk manager, Lauren Thornton, and I were complaining about the malpractice risk environment over an afternoon cup of coffee in the snack bar (doubtless combatting the 4 p. m. nadir) when she shows me an old court transcript she has unearthed.

"Seems one of our revered pediatricians, Dr. Sam Minton, was on the stand some thirty years ago," Lauren said, inserting her own comments. "He was serving as an expert witness for the defense in a malpractice case. Had to do with

215

blindness occurring in a toddler. Sam was well known as a wonderful baby doctor but also as a cagey customer before a jury. Here's how it went."

She read aloud. "Doctor, I know you understand that you are to answer only my questions and answer them directly, right?" That was Randolph Evert, easily the most feared plaintiff's attorney in town.

"Objection!" The defense attorney rose. "The witness must be allowed to answer questions in a complete and coherent manner."

"But only my questions, right, your honor?"

"Correct," said the judge. "Objection overruled."

Evert smiled faintly. "Now, Doctor, you are accustomed to treating newborn babies, correct?"

"I am."

"And how many cases of retrolental fibroplasia like this one have you had?"

"None."

"And I'm sure that's because you're such a careful clinician, right?"

"No, sir."

"No? What's this, Doctor? You're not a careful clinician?"

"Yes, sir, I am."

"Then, exactly what do you mean? How is it you haven't had any cases like this one?"

"I guess I've just been lucky."

"Doctor, I have a very serious question for you."

"Yes, sir."

"Do you understand that at this very moment you are under oath?"

"Yes, counsellor. And as I understand it, I'm the only one in the courtroom at this very moment who is."

Evert turned slightly pale, then slightly violet. "Now, Doctor, this is a terrible case. Please let's come to a focus. This baby was premature, weighed only 5 1/2 pounds at birth, right?"

"Right."

"Now then, tell us what retrolental fibroplasia is."

"It's a gradual accumulation of fibrous tissue inside the eyes. Occurs occasionally in newborns, leads to total blindness within months to years. Occurred more often in preemies."

"And that's what this baby has been suffering with?"

"According to the records I've been given."

"And, doctor, is the cause of this condition known?"

"Yes."

"And," Evert turned, imperiously sweeping his hand before the jury, "exactly what is that cause?"

"High-flow oxygen given during the newborn period."

"And, doctor, did this child receive high-flow oxygen?" Evert was facing the jury now.

"According to the record."

"Then, doctor, would you say that this child's permanent lifetime blindness, due to retrolental fibroplasia, resulted from high-flow oxygen given because the attending physician ordered it?"

217

"Yes."

"And, doctor, do you know that Dr. Mobley, there, was the attending physician?" Evert pointed to the defense table.

"That's what the record shows."

"So this child will go through life denied the gift of vision because of Dr. Mobley's order?"

"Yes."

"No further questions." A faint smile broke through Evert's supercilious expression as he sat down.

"But I have further answers," said Dr. Sam.

"I'm through examining the witness, your honor," said Evert.

"Yes, Dr. Minton. Did you not finish answering the questions?"

Sam faced the judge. "If the court please, I didn't get to the important part."

"Objection!" cried Evert. "I'm finished with this witness!"

"Overruled," said the judge. "I want to hear this. Proceed, Dr. Minton."

Sam turned back to face the gallery, but making sure the jury could hear him. "Your honor, at the time this child was born -- 1959 -- nobody in the world knew that oxygen caused retrolental fibroplasia."

"Objection! Witness is wandering afield."

"Overruled. Doctor, please continue."

Sam went on. "Doctors wondered if it was prematurity, or low birth-weight. Then, in 1963, high-flow

218

oxygen was found to be the culprit. So it made sense that premature and small babies were the ones more likely to get the oxygen, more likely to get retrolental fibroplasia. But since then, there have been no cases of retrolental fibroplasia at U. S. hospitals. A wonderful advance.

"Nobody, not Dr. Mobley, not me, not the pediatricians at Harvard or Johns Hopkins, or anywhere knew about the oxygen thing in 1959. If any of those doctors -- Dr Mobley, or me, or those at the University medical centers -- in 1959 had *failed* to give oxygen to this small premature child, then *that* would have been malpractice on that date, not the reverse. Unfortunate outcome. But Dr. Mobley did the right thing at that time."

I tell you there was a really huge silence in the courtroom.

Then the judge spoke. "Attorney for the defense?

"No redirect examination, your honor."

"They say the jury were out only eight minutes," Lauren said. "They found in favor of Dr. Mobley."

"Dr. Minton said he looked around for the plaintiff's attorney, Randolph Evert, but apparently he had been the first to leave the courtroom."

THE NITTY-GRITTY

I walk back into Room 458 East. "Okay, Dan. Truth time. You were here two weeks ago under an assumed name, not in Arkansas. You begged for shots. Nothing was found. You left without permission when the shots stopped. You

219

aren't enrolled in State Tech. There is no Dr. Madison. Your mother is nowhere to be found."

"Doctor, you mean you don't believe me?"

"Dan, how bad is your habit? What's your drug of choice? How long have you been hooked? What's the dosage level now? Maybe I can get you some help."

He begins sobbing and turns, burying his head in the pillow. Then he surfaces again. "I'm an addict all right, Doctor. A hopeless addict. First pot, then heroin, a little coke, now morphine, Dilaudid, Demerol. Morphine's the cheapest, but Dilaudid's easier to find on the street. Lately I've been taking 10 milligrams of Dilaudid every 3-4 hours."

Ten milligrams. Five times the full analgesic dose. Enough to kill a full-size adult. Respiratory depression would occur in anyone who had built no tolerance. The piddling doses we have been giving Dan have been doing nothing but preventing a full-scale withdrawal syndrome.

"Are you ready for some help?"

"Oh, yes--I've got to have some help. Can you do something for me? I'll agree to anything."

Anything, that is, to stay out of jail, get his regular doses, eventually get back to the street circuit. I'll call in a psychiatrist who does addiction work. He'll try to get him hospitalized in a public facility, since Dan has no funds or insurance. What he needs is a month of inpatient detoxification and education and a lifetime of follow-up. But what will he get? He'll end up at an outpatient treatment center. They'll fool with him awhile, give him some daily methadone. He'll drop out as soon as he can set up a connection. When the money or the connection gives out, he'll try another trick -- another kidney stone, another acute abdomen, another inpatient admission.

But I call the ER, the admitting office, the business office, the record room, outpatient registration. There will be a next time all right-- when the ER staff and the doctors and the administrators are fooled.

But the next time won't be at this hospital.

Poor Dan.

SYMPHONY, ANYONE?

I look at my watch as I crank up the aging BMW in my sub-basement parking spot. The watch says 6:55. The BMW balks. Never got that cold starter kit installed. You can't just take a half-day off to go to the service department out in the boondocks. Of course, the new car department, where you can spend forty or fifty thousand dollars, they put right within walking distance.

Maybe, just maybe, we can make the symphony. Trouble is, if you're a little late they won't let you in. You sit and wait for intermission. Come to think of it, that's not all bad because Tchaikovsky's D Major Violin Concerto with Olivieri playing is after admission anyway, and that's the main event. Matter of fact, it's one of the greatest pieces of music ever written, says I. Every man a judge, every man an expert. Every man to his own taste. *De gustibus non disputandum est.* About the only Latin I remember.

Too bad we had to cancel tennis tonight. The Over-the-Hill Gang -- composed of four physicians in their mid-fifties -- usually gathers on Thursday evenings at The Town Club for an hour and a half of what has been viewed by some as less-than-championship doubles competition. The action is not too fast; in fact, one wry onlooker has described it from a spectator's point of view as frankly restful. A young woman likened it to badminton. The rules, too, are simpler than at Wimbledon. They are dictated by Dr. Fred Wharton, the general surgeon, whose authority in this matter is never questioned. Indeed, Wharton's rules supersede, for this event, those of the American Lawn Tennis Association, but they are enunciated with an air of authority not one whit less confident than the Marquis of Queensbury:

1) the set is over when any team gets to six games (i.e., no tie-breakers -- 6 to 5 may be the final score of the set);

2) the progression is by round-robin, sequence decided by Wharton;

3) three sets are projected, but the play is over at nine-thirty, no matter what, so that there is time for two drinks. Some of us have also suggested that other, unwritten, Whartonian principles are actually in force:

a) questionable line calls are decided by the loudest voice;

b) reaching over the net is permitted if you hit a winner;

c) foot faults are never penalized -- indeed, are never noticed;

d) comments can be made freely about misshits except for Wharton's shots, many of which fall in this category anyway;

e) any fill-in guest never pays for his drinks but must be careful not to play too well if he wishes a rematch.

At the end, the "good CD" (winning Common Denominator) and bad CD (loser) are identified, and blame and credit are appropriately assigned. For example, Wharton always seems to find his partners deficient, even though they are the same partners everyone else had. Once a guest ended up as the good CD. Not only was he not issued another invitation, no one spoke to him during the post-mortem session. As I remember, he only got one drink. But he had his revenge: he ordered Glenfiddich on the rocks at $12.00 a shot.

But it is not the tennis(?) nor the innuendo nor the drinks which make weekly attendance mandatory at this event. It is not even the obligatory jokes at the commencement of the social portion of the program which impel these busy physicians to desert their patients or their dinner-tables to migrate, like lemmings, to the Town Club.

It is the gossip. Norman did it again, says Harmon Jackson, the radiologist. He came in, demanded some films, exploded because they weren't already pulled, chewed out the film clerk, raised hell with the director of technologists, had three girls crying before he left. Got to talk to him about that. Hear it's the same way in the operating room. If they don't have a certain retractor, or it had to be re-autoclaved, it hits the fan. He throws various other tools around, prowls around

223

the operating table, yells, scrub nurses rip off their masks, leave the operating room. One quit last week, just walked out of the hospital with her scrub dress still on, crying.

"That's bad," I put in, "but that's only because he's an impatient perfectionist. What's really bad is what happened last week. I'm talking about Carl Simpson. Being chief of medicine would be a snap for me without him around. He admitted a patient to the regular floor with chest pain. That's fine. Then he went up and took some more history. That's good, too. After further discussion, he apparently decided her pain was suggestive enough of a myocardial infarction that she'd be better off in the coronary care unit. That's OK, no problem, good thinking. But then there was a delay in transfer so decided to move her himself. They didn't have a bed in the CCU, so the nurses had to get permission to move someone out. That took a little time. But that's not the punch line of the story."

I can tell I've got their attention now. Drinks are put down, hands are folded, heads are inclined my way.

"What is the punch line?" asks Harmon, the radiologist.

"The punch line is, he walked her out of the hospital to his car and took her to another hospital. Four miles. Where it would take hours to get her into a bed. Lady with a possible heart attack. In front of the nurses. Even the orderlies dropped their teeth."

"Did you talk to him?" Samuel, the hematologist-internist, wants to know.

"Talk to him, sure. Didn't make a dent."

"What in God's name did he say?"

"Said she didn't have a heart attack anyway."

"But for Christ's sake he moved her, suspecting she did."

"Right. I mentioned that. He said they were slow in getting her moved. I said what was the rush."

"And then what did he say?" Now Wharton is in on the action.

"He said she was too critical to wait."

"So what the hell did you say then, John?"

"I told him the next time he pulled something like this he wouldn't have to talk to me about it. He said that was good, he wasn't learning anything from me anyway."

"Then what?" Wharton is really attentive now.

"I said, you won't be talking to me, you'll be talking to the Hospital Board."

But, as I say, tennis was cancelled tonight; work occasionally interferes. There are two beeps on the way home and then I remember -- stop at the supermarket. Mary Alice practically never assigns me this job, so I can't complain.

KROGER DIAGNOSIS

Furthermore, I don't actually mind going to the supermarket with a real mission -- for example, buying for a whole meal. Matter of fact I read in a survey that the power and glory conferred upon the housewife by spending $200 for the family's seven-day ration is the high point of the week, complain though she will. On the other hand it is a pain to get three items and wait in line, stand and freeze next to the dairy counter. But here I am-- the responsibility for a pound of oleo, one half-gallon of milk, and one-quarter pound of sugar vested in my dubious hands. The elderly man in front of me apparently is here for the night, and it's getting colder and colder here by the refrigerated goods. No way to make the first half of the symphony.

Then I see her. She is overweight. Her face is puffy. The skin has a curious shiny, lemon-yellow hue -- no, more orange, like a bleached carrot. She moves very slowly; she almost creeps. Age? Maybe 28, 30. She sits down as if to wait for someone. Her features, on closer scrutiny, are coarse, almost Oriental. No, the coarseness is due to edema, swelling. Her head swings from side to side no faster than a turtle. Though I admit this supermarket is chilly, it is a warm October, the outside temperature is 64 -- and she has on a long-sleeved blouse, a sweater, and a windbreaker!

Of course, this is none of my business. Nothing could be more inappropriate than what I now will do. I walk up, pay for my paltry purchases, pick up my amateurish sack, pass through the register area, and then go to the manager's booth.

"Pardon me, ma'am, but have you ever seen that young woman before?"

"Well, yes, she's been in here several times," says the perky lady. She shakes the hair out of her face. "Always comes with an older woman, maybe her mother. May I ask why you want to know, sir?" A trace, just a trace of suspicion crosses the manager's face.

"Yes, well, I'm a doctor, and I happened to notice her. I believe she's got a problem."

"Why, I do too, now that you mention it. Something strange about her."

"Thanks a lot." Diagnosticians everywhere. They call me all day: Bill needs a cholesterol, Doctor, and a mono test wouldn't be a bad idea -- he's been so tired. I don't want to be an interfering mother but will you do a drug screen and an AIDS test on Julia? Sandy must have something wrong with his hormones -- can you check that out or does he need to see an endocrinologist? And now the Kroger manager is carrying out clinical investigation. And doing a pretty good job.

I decide that time's a-wastin', so I go right up to the girl and extend my hand. "Hello, Winifred, how are you?"

The pause is breathtakingly long. She surveys me like an owl. She says nothing for what seems one eon. Then, as if in slow motion, she puts out her hand. Her voice can only be described as croaking.

"I'm -- not -- Winifred -- I'm Vir-ginia." Her hand is cadaverously cold, slick, like a chilled pigskin glove.

I shake her hand and apologize. "I thought sure you were someone else. Glad to meet you anyway, Virginia." Big smile. I withdraw my hand and she won't let go. And won't let go. *And won't let go!* Finally, she releases my fingers and, in slow motion again, returns her hand to her side.

A middleaged woman comes up and smiles at Virginia. "Who is this, dear?"

227

"I'm sorry. My name is Dr. John Galen and I'm afraid I have mistaken Virginia for somone else named Winifred. Are you Virginia's older sister (I'm beginning to learn things in my old age)?

"No, her mother, but thanks."

"Could I speak to you a moment?"

We walk to the other side of the array of wire wheelcarts. " Mrs.--"

"Janson."

"Mrs. Janson. This is strictly none of my business, but as I say I happen to be a physician and I must ask you: Has Virginia has been to a doctor recently?"

"Well, no, not in a good many years. Why?"

"Have you noticed any change in her lately?

"Yes, sleeps a lot, no energy, cold all the time. And some -- some other things."

"Constipation? Heavy menstrual periods?"

"Why, yes, how did you, how could you --"

"Mrs. Janson, I would be very, very suspicious of thyroid deficiency in your daughter. I mean severe hypothyroidism. I just couldn't walk by without suggesting you get it checked. Pretty easy to diagnose and very easy to treat. Might make a lot of difference in her life."

"Why, we will -- look into it. Thank you -- thank you very much."

I turn to go.

"Doctor--"

"Yes?"

"What did you say your name was?"

228

The Lone Ranger is on my lips but I resist. "Galen. John Galen."

"Thank you again."

Back in the BMW again, sputtering again, for the space of 1.1 miles to my house, I consider the question of the thyroid gland. Master controller of metabolism, the little hourglass-shaped blob of flesh in the front of the neck dictates the pace of life. Overactive, it will drive the heart at a terrific clip, make the hands vibrate, speed up the bowels, smooth out the skin, cause weight loss. Underactive, you have Virginia: drowsy, slow-moving, overweight, mentally obtunded, puffy, weak, constipated, undoubtedly sexually retarded. She is cold all the time and so are her hands. The muscles are slow to move and slower to relax. Point is, a few blood tests confirm this diagnosis, and treatment is child's play, consisting these days of a synthetic thyroid hormone replacement, the dose being titrated to an optimal level. A tablet a day. Sometimes, as here, the condition is missed: the family doesn't notice the day-to-day change. Even the family doctor may be lulled by the imperceptible progress of the disease: week by week, year by year, he doesn't notice. Indeed, the diagnosis may elude the consultant if he doesn't think of it immediately. Somewhere along the line, though, the constellation of signs and symptoms will break through the glassy surface of a doctor's consciousness like a rising pike. *Splash!* Diagnosis suspected, confirmed. *Blink!* Patient treated. Quality of human life restored. If you're the doctor, can you resist? The child in the burning building, the dog baking in the closed car: can you just walk on by?

MARY ALICE SAYS

As I pull in the little circular drive in front of our not-very-pretentious but solidly built 60-year-old English cottage, I speculate on what Mary Alice will be doing at the moment. This woman, my auburn-haired and green-eyed bride of 35 years, is not a lady with tentative opinions. Though she may at times cash in on her womanly privilege to be ambivalent, she does not spend much time roiling around in the grey limbo between black and white. Furthermore, the range of subjects on which she has not reached firm conclusions is small indeed. At her last birthday party, she was given the EB Award for making it unnecessary to keep an Encyclopedia Brittanica around. I have always felt that a detailed psychological analysis of Mary Alice would result in a perfect score for mental hygiene -- she has never experienced guilt from repressing a thought.

The patients love her -- indeed, I have suspected they call at night asking for a prescription refill but really with the hope of talking to Mary Alice.   While she carefully avoids giving any medical advice she does not hesitate to provide counsel on virtually any other subject: "Honey, don't put up with that kind of stuff from your husband -- tell him to shape up or ship out. He won't leave, he'll love you for it." "That's a better school, anyway, with a lot better class of students." "That's the secret -- don't put in too much yeast but give it plenty of time to rise."

230

Mary Alice, you see, got me through medical training in the first place. Not paid my way, exactly – we scraped by on the GI Bill, on my hand-to-mouth advertising business on the side, and a lot of luck. But she fed the children grits, fixed everything that broke herself, stretched each nickel until it screamed. Naturally prudent, anyway, she saw to it that we didn't actually *take* a newspaper. We had a five-party telephone line. She washed the paper plates, saved up remnant shreds of soap, melted them down, cut them up into new bars. She still picks up ice dropped on the floor and puts it in the house plants to save water.

As I started my first year in medical school, she set a new record. She was pregnant with our second-born and we were trying to make our new little house livable, so she wanted to plan ahead.

"What kind of sandwich do you like best for lunch?" she asked.

"I guess creamed-cheese-and-chopped-olive," I replied, innocently.

She came in one day with a case of creamed cheese and a small vat of green olives. Soon I discovered that our moderate-sized freezer chest was chock-a-block with small tightly folded brown paper sacks. Each contained two creamed-cheese-etc. sandwiches. Each morning I would find a metal instrument and carefully chip out one unit. Then, arriving at medical school, I would position the sack on the seat so it would catch the full rays of the sun and thaw by lunch. Sometimes you would have to sneak out and move the sack as the sun rose higher.

231

The children actually had a fairly easy life; that is, they didn't have to loll around wondering what they should be doing (she had already told them) or what they could get away with (basically nothing, she had already thought of it). They are now, of course, perfect. All because of her.

So what will she be up to now? Let's see:

1. She'll be on the telephone (in which activity she has a black belt).

2. She'll be watching MCN, the Money Cable Network (the stock market is an area of her real expertise).

3. She'll have a neighbor over for counselling (they stand in line to see what Mary Alice Says).

4. She has just finished retouching one of her still lifes or landscapes, her late-discovered talent a wonder to all.

She meets me at the door. "Can't you ever be on time?" (This from one who has never even been close.)

"Sorry, Sugar. You know how it is."

"Yes, I know how it is. It is, that at eight o'clock they won't even let us *in* the symphony."

"Patients, you know."

"Patience, hell. All I have is patience."

"I mean *patients. ts,* not *ce.* Certain patients you just can't leave -- you know, until they're taken care of."

EMERGENCY?

At 7:21 p. m., the beeper is insistent: MRS. M. ROBERTSON - EMERGENCY - MRS. M. ROBERTSON - 350-1521 - EMERGENCY

Two thoughts surface. First is Galen's' Rule: Any *routine* page may signify any of a range of problems from the most trivial to the most urgent and disastrous -- from an early head cold to a heart attack -- but an *emergency* page is *never* an emergency. The Rule has, to my memory, remained sacrosanctly inviolate. Just out of a morbid curiosity, I have frequently asked people, after dealing with the headache, or the house guest's turned ankle, just why they decided to ask the operator to designate the call "emergency." The answers are revealing: "Well, we're going out of town in the morning, and I wanted to make sure we got a refill before the drugstores closed -- they close early on Sunday night, you know." Or "I was afraid we wouldn't be able to get you with a routine call, since this was just about an appointment." (I've never figured that one out at all.) "Well, I know it's not really an emergency, but I was getting ready to go to the movie and couldn't wait. And, Doctor -- I didn't want to bother you at the office." (I'm not sure whether that involves a non-sequitur or an undistributed middle term.)

The Uncontested Winner, though, was this one:

CALL LYNN ENGSTROM - EMERGENCY - LYNN ENGSTROM - 355-3933 - EMERGENCY

"Ms. Engstrom? Dr. Galen. "What is it?"

"Oh, Doctor, thanks so much for calling. I thought I'd better get the answer to this right away and not wait. How quickly do birth control pills work?"

"Well, usually they will prevent the next ovulation if you start two weeks ahead of time. A month is safer."

"Oh. Well, what if, like, somebody was going to have intercourse. Would starting the pills now help?"

"Not if you were already ovulating. If you're not ovulating, then of course, it would be safe anyway. When are you and your husband actually, er, planning to have intercourse?"

"Well, not exactly my husband, you know. It's more like my fiance."

"Okay. Well, when will you and -- your fiance--"

"We're not exactly sure."

"Oh."

"That is, we're not exactly sure when we'll *finish*. Uh. Oh. Uh. I mean, should I take it now or wait till it's --uh, oh -- over?"

"Lynn, under the circumstances, why don't you just wait til it's over."

The second thought that swims over from the right side of my brain, in the process of answering Mrs. Robertson's call, is this question: Why is she phoning now when I just left her -- and her very sick husband -- ten minutes ago?

A call to Mrs. Robertson in her husband's hospital room fails to throw light on this question: "He's just going downhill, Dr. Galen. Getting worse all the time. And nobody's doing anything."

"Well, now, Emma, you know we've talked about this over and over. You know he has cancer everywhere. Everybody agrees that further radiation or chemotherapy wouldn't help -- in fact, would hurt him. Dr. Franklin agrees.

234

M. D. Anderson agrees. Sloan-Kettering agrees. I agree. You and your son and Martin's brother agree. We all want to keep him comfortable. And we're doing everything we can to accomplish that."

"Yes, but he's not comfortable. He's breathing heavily."

"He was asleep a few minutes ago. Has he waked up?"

"Well, no."

"If he's asleep I doubt if he's aware of any discomfort. I guess that's all we can ask."

"All right, Dr. Galen. Thank you."

7:25 p. m. MRS. ROBERTSON - EMERGENCY - 350-1521 - MRS ROBERTSON - EMERGENCY.

"Dr. Galen, nobody's doing anything. The nurses are terrible. They won't do lift a hand. I had to fire one today."

"Yes, Emma. And you fired one yesterday and two the day before."

"The floor nurses aren't interested at all."

"Now, now. They're some of the best we've got. You remember you wanted to move up from 3 Center because you didn't like the personnel down there."

"Maybe we'd better move back."

"No, Emma, I think we'd better stick with what we're doing."

Again, and again, and then again--a total of seven emergency pages in an hour. I think I know the problem, and I think I can't handle it over the phone.

"I'll drop you by the symphony, Sugar, and join you at intermission."

"Not interested in going to the symphony alone -- not that interested in the symphony anyway." Her cheeks seem to develop the same auburn color as her hair. "Who is it -- Mrs. Robertson again? Hasn't she fired you yet?"

"No, but she's kicked everybody else off the case -- nurses, oncologists, urologists."

"Wonder what she sees in you."

"That's one way to look at it. Guess she has to keep one doctor around in order to authorize Mr. Robertson being in the hospital -- and to have somebody to ventilate at."

"She's crazy."

"In a way. She feels crazy right now. I'll have to go talk to her."

"Gonna' push the right button and straighten everything out in a few minutes?"

"No, but I may be able to put my finger on the right nerve."

"I hope it's her finger nerve -- the one that dials telephones. Good luck. I'll be right here. We'll have to go after intermission. I'll fix something to eat."

Mrs. Robertson is pacing the floor near the nursing station. Her brow is furrowed, her eyes frantic. She periodically moves as if to run her fingers through -- but ends up only caressing -- the lateral masses of her newly coiffed hair.

"Let's go have a look," I say, trying to exude enough *aequanimitas* to please the famous Dr. Osler. At the bedside, with chart in hand, I see nothing to suggest a change in Mr. Robertson's condition. He is asleep. The oxygen tube is in place across his upper lip. It sends branching tusks into his nasal passages, hissing out the essential vapor in 100 percent concentration to mix with the room air in his nasopharynx; his lungs end up with 30-40 percent, substantially more than the 20 percent available in the Earth's atmosphere. His vital signs remain normal. This respiration, to be sure, is a little heavy, almost stertorous; but this is unchanged and is, furthermore, only what one would expect in a man whose lungs are peppered with metastases from his cancer of the kidney, called renal cell carcinoma. In addition, the tumor involves his spine, his liver, and is spread around the abdominal cavity. All this is evident from conventional x-rays, bone scans, CT scans. Moreover, his liver involvement is obvious on palpating his abdomen; the organ, normally firm and barely perceptible below the rib cage, is in Mr. Robertson's case large, hard, and studded with rocky irregularities.

Once, again, I examine Mr. Robertson in some detail -- not with much of a rational medical indication, for there is no change from the similar exam one hour ago -- but as a basis for the educational program I am now formulating for his wife.

"He's getting worse every minute," she cries out, causing him to stir slightly. "The nurses won't come when I call."

"Now, Emma, Miss Tucker just walked out as we came in."

"That's the first in a long time -- she must have known you were coming."

"Does she know you don't have private-duty nurses now? That you let the last one go about an hour ago?"

Mrs. Robertson drops her hands to her sides, frustration showing. "I don't know, Dr. Galen, I don't know."

"Let's go down to the lounge and go over everything, Emma." I know that proposing a conference gives the proposer the upper hand. He is the comptroller of the situation -- that is, if he has anything substantive to say. And I don't want to forget Joan Rivers.

The open lounge has comfortable chairs and sofas, and several windows give out upon the remaining forests of the northwest portion of the city.

"Emma, you know the situation. Martin is near the end. He's in no distress. He gets morphine for the least discomfort. He's on oxygen. There's nothing else to do. Everybody agrees. He's getting excellent care. But then we're having a problem, aren't we? -- a big one. Nurses and doctors are getting fired. His wife is pacing the floor. I answer seven emergency calls in an hour. I come back up here. Nothing is wrong with the management of the patient. What's the trouble, then?"

Emma shakes her head.

"You don't know?"

"No."

"I think I know, Emma."

"Well, what, Doctor, what?"

"I think the problem quite honestly is with you. Experience shows that when a family member has great distress and starts complaining about everything, agitating about, even though the patient is being well handled, the problem is the family member's attitude."

"I just want Martin to get good treatment. But you say attitude?"

"Yes. Most of the time in situations like this it turns out that the relative has a load of guilt about the person who is dying. And guilt is hard to bear. People will do anything to get rid of it. They will shift it to someone else -- anyone: doctors, nurses, aides, other family members. Emma, look at me and listen: do you feel guilty about Martin for any reason?"

She gasps, covers her mouth, gazes out the window, drops her hand again, leaves her mouth agape. "Guilty? Guilty? Me?" She looks at me and again out the window. She clasps her head with both hands, then returns them to her lap. "I don't think so, I mean, I shouldn't be. I mean, just those few times I went on trips without him. He didn't like cruises anyway. And you know those little shipboard romances don't amount to anything, do they? I mean, sex is just sex and. . . ." Emma bursts into tears.

"It's not a matter of whether you should be guilty or not -- it's whether you *feel* guilty," I point out. You actually have been a good wife, and Martin thinks so. Here you are, doing everything you can. I'm not interested in your Love Boat capers and neither is Martin."

At this moment her son, a dentist, and his wife walk off the elevator.

"Oh, John," Emma says. "Your father is much worse. They won't do anything. I've had to fire the nurses again. Dr. Galen is the only doctor we've got left, the only one we can keep on the case, and now he comes and says that everything is fine and I'm just causing an uproar. Can you believe that?"

"I'm sure Dr. Galen doesn't mean it quite that way, Mother."

"I never said everything is fine, Emma," I put in. "You know that. Nothing is fine. Everything is bad. I just think you're unnecessarily upset. Let's talk more tomorrow, and you think about some of the things I've said."

She will think, and we shall talk, but the guilt is there and the problem will remain. It is a familiar scene at the hospital nursing station: the irate family member, complaining about everything and nothing. The IV is not working, the oxygen is too low, or too high, the patient's not getting any attention, the food's awful, the medication is not working, it must be the wrong drug. Nurses try to reassure, things get worse, then the nurses get abused, get upset. Sometimes the family member requests a transfer to another floor.

It's a lot easier when you understand. The troublemaker is not the daughter who has assiduously cared for the ailing parent, not the loving spouse. It's the son from out of town who has carefully avoided responsibility for the sick subject -- usually for years. Now he's going to expiate his remorse by levying demands on others -- as if to say, I'm

240

going to show you that it's not me that's reneged on my responsibilities and my love. It's you -- you're the one who's at fault.

But nobody's at fault exactly. Martin is dying. And Emma needs relief. I'll give it to her, as much as she'll let me, one small vial at a time.

A LITTLE NIGHT MUSIC

Walking from the parking lot to the Hall, I note the beeps have grown to four -- still routine calls. Now it's the calls versus the first movement of the Tchaikovsky, live, by a world-class violinist.

I hook the beeper back on my belt.

Tchaikovsky wins.

It starts again as Olivieri completes the first movement at 9:15. Buzz-buzz. . . buzz-buzz . . . a slow volley mounting to a salvo. Fortunately the new pager-telephone holds 40 messages in its LED display system, including names and phone numbers. And it's on vibrate, not ring. (One patient, recently single, told me her only excitement in life was to set her cell phone on vibrate, put in in her pocket, and have friends call her.)

On the telephone in the inconvenient and noisy lobby of the high-ceilinged hall, I talk to Mrs. Miller about her postherpetic neuralgia which has hung on ever since the shingles five weeks ago. We're doing all we can, ma'am. . . gabapentin, etc. I wish there were some magic, give it time. Indeed I wish there was something more for these unfortunate

241

people, usually the older ones like Mrs. Miller, who have suffered nerve damage from the inconsiderate virus of *Herpes zoster,* and in whom the pain may persist for months, even for all their days.

Mr. Donald says his chest pain went away so quickly after that nitroglycerine that now he's worried it might be his heart. Aren't those heart medicines? Yes, but we used it here to relax your esophagus, Mr. Donald, just as we discussed day before yesterday. Guess Mr. D. was listening to some other voice while I elaborated on the various actions of those drugs and told him his heart was sound. (I have to think of the lady who accompanied her flushed, red-nosed husband in for reports on his physical. He told both of us that he did his own thing, and then she asked if it was possible that this different drummer he marched to, by any chance, owned a distillery?)

No, Mr. Andrus, don't eat anything in the morning before your stress test. And don't take any medications before you go (just like it says on the sheet you're looking at, and just as Sandra told you). And I know the real reason you called, Mr. Andrus. I hope my voice tells you: this test is not going to be dangerous, it's carefully monitored.

BEEP BEEP . . . BEEP BEEP . . .PAGE # 8 -- EMERGENCY ROOM METRO HOSP -654-3333 -- NURSE JOAN

BEEP BEEP . . . BEEP BEEP . . .PAGE # 9 -- EMERGENCY ROOM METRO HOSP --654-3334 -- NURSE MARCIE.

So they're not talking to each other down there tonight. Sometimes I serve as a human intercom.

"Marcie? Joan? Oh, Ruth. John Galen. Can I speak to Marcie or Joan? Or maybe you want me too? Never mind . . ." There is a clatter and some yelling in the background.

"Dr. Galen? Marcie. We don't know what to do with this one. Big as a beached whale and he can't move. Says he's a kidney patient of yours. Short of breath tonight and weaker. Now seems paralyzed. Vitals aren't that good. Blood pressure 70 systolic, and that's only by Doppler. Pulse 47, Respiration shallow at 32 per minute. Name's Randolph Brown."

Randolph. Forty-eight years old. Chronic glomerulonephritis. Progressive kidney failure, holding his own on diet, meds. Doing fairly well two weeks ago in the office. Now -- big trouble.

"Get an EKG, portable chest, lytes, gases, start some D-5-W, nasal O2 at three liters. He might have hyperkalemia."

"We've done all that. Nothing back yet. Hyper - what?

"Potassium. His potassium may have shot up."

"Up? Does that make you weak? I thought *down* made you weak."

"Both. This sounds more like up than down. Is that cardiogram ready?"

"Uh -- here it comes."

"What do the QRS complexes look like?"

"Let's see . . .kind of broad, like maybe point twelve."

243

"Uh-oh. What about the T waves?"

"Sorta, like, sharp. Peaked."

"Uh-huh. And the P waves?"

"They're flat, in some leads you can't see them. PR interval is real long."

"OK. We've got to assume hyperK while we wait for the lab. You got an ER doctor?"

"Two of them. Both up to their necks in alligators in the trauma rooms. Talk to me -- and can you come?"

"I'm coming, I'm coming.   But I'm fifteen minutes away. Do about five things -- are you ready?"

"I'm ready."

"Give him two amps of soda bicarb. Fifty ccs of 50% glucose. Ten units of insulin. One amp of calcium gluconate or calcium chloride, either one, I don't care. All IV push. Stat. Then put calcium in the drip -- what is it, 1000 cc?

"I'm looking . . . it's . . . 500."

"OK. Two amps of calcium in that bag.   And run it at 100 an hour. Then Kayexalate -- give him a 60-cc bottle of that Kayexalate-sorbitol mixture p. o. Got all that?"

She repeats everything, in detail, without the doctor-slang and then asks, "Right?"

"Right."

Marcie's voice gets muffled. "Anne, get on this right now. I know, I know, don't worry about that cast right now." Back into the mouthpiece, "Anything else?"

"Yeah, leave him hooked up to the monitor so we can follow his pattern. And thanks for straightening me out."

"For what?"

"For correcting my slang."

"Correcting doctors -- that's a nurse's job."

"OK, now can I speak to Joan?"

"Yes, I think she's got a stroke for you."

ALUMNI, ALUMNAE

As we drive away from Symphony Hall, where we finally caught the last half of the concerto, but not the last number, the pager beeps twice, but I contain my curiosity until we arrive at home.

On call. It's no bargain.

Last Thursday night was better, but not much. I remember it in detail.

I arrived at the Jones University Medical Alumni cocktail-dinner-meeting late. Not because of saving lives but because I had first gone to the wrong building on campus. Got to speak to Natalie about that. After all, she is in charge of programming my schedule -- her phrasing is "changing my diapers." Soon we were congregated in the sun room of a beautiful old converted residence donated to the University by a patron. In situations like this you should act as if you are used to such luxus ambience. Everybody else was acting that way, too.

I shook hands with a lot of old friends from medical school and training days. I hadn't seen them since last year, when almost the identical group was here for the executive board meeting. It's always the same ones who do this work. We all feel slightly superior and slightly martyred by these contributions to community endeavor, secretly suspecting that

245

all the others are selfishly off recreating or making money. Even more secretly, some of us may admit at least to ourselves that we need the ego-uplift of such pseudo-honorific positions. Financially non-remunerative though they may be, these titular appointments fuel the furnace of a self-esteem which is daily doused by perhaps the same thousand natural shocks which Hamlet complained of.

Indeed, it is the physician's lot to be beset by this very psychopathology. Every study that is done confirms it: the MD has to earn his emotional wings every day. If you're a doctor, every time you wake up you have *carte blanche* -- not in the popular sense of unlimited privilege, but in the classic Locke/Berkeley/Hume sense of blank sheet. Each morning you start over, proving yourself again and again. The physician prescribes restoratives for the patient; the patient himself is the restorative for the physician. The grateful smile is addicting. You want it again and again, cannot get enough, will drive yourself to obtain that craved potion. You are the rat whose tiny midbrain is invaded by the miniature electrode, implanted strategically in the pleasure center. The rat presses the pedal and experiences the malaise, releases it and feels the euphoria. Press it again! Release! Ah! You are the drug addict (somewhat like Dan Godwick) who is the victim not so much of physiological dependency, but a pawn of the experience itself. Feel that intense intellectual excitement, feel it recede, and you must have it again! You, and Coleridge, and Sherlock Holmes. If, like the cocaine freak, you have a small empty place in your spiritual anatomy; if you are not quite whole but must fill the vacuum daily -- who knows, you may become a doctor, my son. Soon this vacuum will fill, and fill again, and then demand filling. It will become a black hole in your soul, sucking up human gratitude with insatiable gravitational force. You will do your work with secret rapture. You will complain about your hours, to be sure, but with tongue firmly embedded in cheek. You will groan loudly about inadequate reimbursement for cognitive services and government intervention and DRGs and HMOs. But you will carefully never admit to the authorities what every true physician-addict knows so well: you would pay to do this.

Like the heroin devotee, the magnitude of one's ensnarement in this scenario is best gauged by a trial of withdrawal. The true intravenous drug abuser will become mortally ill upon cessation of his daily dose -- may indeed succumb. The authentic physician, on reaching his vacation site, will become a pacing jungle animal. It is not merely boredom that besets him. Deprived of his essential sequence of pressure, demand, and gratification, his pupils dilate and his *joie de vivre* is supplanted by an *angor animi*: it is more than he can bear. He now must water-ski or snow-ski or climb a barely climbable mountain or at the very minimum achieve exhaustion with tennis or golf. So critically in demand is a structured formula for this dread week that several magazines are dedicated to providing survival schemes for the physician's vacation. *Escape* and *Getaway* are two of them. Plan enough glittering distractions and perhaps you will live through it. You ravenously hunger for such deliverance until you get there. And then, and then -- at the end of the week -- there is always the longed-for relief. The return to nirvana.

Back to work.

"Don't know what we'd do without you good people," said the new Dean. "You're a nucleus we hope to build on."

Everybody is always building, moving, climbing. Stop for a minute and the juggernaut of old debt, old commitments will crush you. Run, keep running. Don't look back, said Satchel, and the administrators have taken up the philosophy.

Just as dinner was announced the beeper went off -- right on schedule (notice how I have learned to complain reflexly). I excused myself and found, on the foyer telephone, that Mrs. Cefalu was reluctant to surrender the floor, even though it was Mr. Cefalu who is having the rectal bleeding.

"What color is the blood, Mrs. Cefalu?"

"Just a minute." Long pause. Distant conversation. "Red."

"Bright red?"

"Just a minute." Another long interval. "Yes, he thinks so."

"How much?"

"What?"

"May I speak to Mr. Cefalu?" I asked more loudly. There was another pause. The soft pulse of conversation went on in the next room. Mr. Cefalu, alas, was deafer than the Mrs. "HOW MUCH BLOOD IS IT?"

"What?"

I repeated the question, still louder.

"Not too much."

"DOES IT SEEM TO BE COMING FROM HEMORRHOIDS?"

"What's that you say?"

The conversation seemed to have died in the next room. I took a deep breath. "ARE YOU SURE IT'S YOUR RECTUM?"

Finally, reasonably convinced that Mr. Cefalu has a minor hemorrhoidal problem, I prescribed warm sitz baths, a stool softener, a witch hazel application, and a lubricant suppository.

I returned to the dining room and found everyone smiling broadly at me. They seemed to be glad I was back. Someone was so glad he began laughing. Then everybody broke up.

I sat down next to the Dean. He was smiling over his salmon mousse.

"What's the joke, Henry?" I asked.

He snickered. "Well, we were saying grace, that is, Dr. Casey was." He continued to look at his salmon mousse.

"Yes."

"Well, actually, Dr. Williams asked Dr. Casey if he even knew a blessing."

"And?"

"And he said he'd have to reach down somewhere and see what he could come up with."

"Go on."

"And then you screamed 'Are you sure it's your rectum?'"

"Oh, God."

"But that wasn't the main thing."

"No?"

"No. The main thing was when Dr. Casey recited ' . . .accept our thanks for these and all thy many other blessings . . ."

"Yes?"

"And before he could say 'Amen' you filled in with 'Tucks pads and glycerin suppositories.'"

HOME AGAIN, BRIEFLY

Driving through city traffic with one possible and one for-real emergency at the other end of the trip would, when I was younger, have presented a dilemma: how fast, how many chances to take? Then over the years I figured it out: if you have a wreck or get stopped by the police you'll be -- tragically -- hours late (the cops aren't impressed that you're a doctor on emergency call anymore: "Sure, Doc. What happened, you get behind from playing golf all afternoon?"). But if you drive carefully, you'll get there only two minutes later than Al Unser. So just stop at the light at the Prado and stay in the middle lane. Left lane is for left turn only. Right lane is for right turn only. And of course everybody's in the center lane. So stay there and cool it.

That's what Mary Alice, my wife of some 40 summers, now riding shotgun in my old BMW, is doing -- being cool, *very* cool.

250

"I don't know why we ever try to go anywhere when you're on call." she says. "It's just a hassle. Don't bother to ask me out again under these conditions."

"Most girls are anxious for dates."

"Not sandwich dates."

"Sandwich? Who's the other party?"

"Miss Jane Beeper. She's grossly impolite, demanding, takes all your attention, interrupts at awkward moments."

"Yeah, and I can't even stand her up."

"Like you do me."

"You've got a point. Tell you what, how about dinner at the club tomorrow night -- I'm definitely off call then."

"And definitely exhausted from tonight."

"You're just hard to get, aren't you?"

"Isn't that what you liked in the first place?"

"That's another point. Want to drop me at the hospital now?"

"No. Take me home. You can have the car all night. But be home by 1 a. m."

"What's 1 a. m.?"

"That's when the TV goes solid hard rock."

"And that's when you need other entertainment?"

"That's when I need to start uninterrupted sleep."

I pull into the circular drive in front of our English cottage. It's not a mansion, but it was built like a fortress during the Great Depression to last many more earth cycles.

I open the car door for Mary Alice. Then the front door of the house.

251

"No goodnight kiss?" I ask.

"What kind of girl do you think I am?"

I ponder this question and stroke my chin. "I guess the word is . . . *different*."

Without changing her mock-severe expression she stands on her tiptoes and kisses me on the forehead.

"That the appetizer?" I ask.

"That, friend, was the entree."

MARY ALICE GOES NORTH

As I walk toward the car, it occurs to me that *different* is indeed a word which applies to my wife. I reflect on our training year in Boston. Mary Alice is a fifth-generation Southern magnolia, and I should have known that efforts to transplant her, even temporarily, to a northern environment would involve a major adjustment reaction. Shortly after arrival, she visited the nearby A&P (they had them then). She asked to speak to the person in charge, then promptly presented him with *a letter of introduction* from her hometown A&P manager. Observing the scene, I at first assumed the man was struck dumb. Then he upgraded his profile by summoning all the employees in the store. They gathered around the cash registers.

"I want all of you to listen," he said, "to this lady talk. It's unique."

"Unique?" said Mary Alice. "Why, I'm the only one here who speaks English. The other customers back there have French or Asian accents."

252

First the small crowd laughed, then they looked at each other, then they applauded.

Shortly thereafter, one of the employees came to the manager and complained she couldn't understand just what Mrs. Galen wanted.

"She keeps saying she wants *grease* or something."

The resourceful manager stepped in. "What was it you wanted, madam?"

"Grits," she said (admittedly *gri-i-i-ts*).

"Oh," said the manager. Is that some type of cereal, maybe made from corn or hominy?"

"Don't tell me you don't know," Mary Alice said. "Grits are Georgia ice cream."

Eventually, the manager set in a supply of grits for Mary Alice, having to fill several shelves with a huge quantity from the importer.

The A&P manager turned out not to be the only executive nonplussed by our heroine in Boston. The local bank director was only momentarily taken aback by the introductory letter from Mary Alice's neighborhood banker. He didn't understand that the author, Mr. Thompson, was an old friend of the family and so this Boston financial officer was taken completely aback by the last sentence:

"And if Mary Alice needs any money at any time, you just let me know."

So I get back into the BMW, which doesn't balk this time. I am sweating a little. About Randolph. I turn on WIN, the classic music station. Mendelssohn's Fifth, the

253

Reformation, is on. I like it. It meets my requirements for a classical symphony: at least three haunting melodies, beautifully developed. Carlo-Menotti said every great melody is buried somewhere in every man's soul, and the composer's job is just to expose it, or words to that effect. I guess Jung would like that oblique reference to the collective unconscious. Anyway, anything without a melody I'm suspicious of. If there's no melody I wonder if the composer can really compose.

It's a lot like cooking. I admit my childhood ill prepared me for *la nouvelle cuisine*, the kind we had at the alumni meeting last week. You spend your formative years eating country-fried steak, catfish, mashed potatoes with gravy, and slabs of unchopped collard greens, and you really don't have the kind of background one needs to enjoy a tiger lily formed from medallions of veal and shoots of scantily cooked legumes. All of which sits in the center of the plate, mind you -- a platter, by the way, which is enormous. The majority of the plate, you see, is empty. In the twenty-first century, apparently, it's rude to fill the plate. My grandmother in 1940 thought it was rude to leave empty spots. Worse, my mother thought playing in one's plate, making designs, was frankly obscene. Yet any *de rigueur* dessert of today surely requires blatant fingerpainting in the kitchen.

Why do they all stop at Peachtree even when the light is green? There's nothing there to hold them up. Maybe they're paying homage to the Old South, which, by the way, there ain't no more of.

Music and dining are actually a lot like art. They kept saying that Picasso was the greatest going, maybe the greatest of all time. I said privately that most of his work which I had seen was ridiculous, what with one-dimensional women facing two ways at once and their breasts pointing at each other. To earn an honest opinion, and to divest myself of my unforgiveable artistic naiveté, I went to the Picasso retrospective at the Museum of Modern Art in New York. There were 1000 originals there, and I stared carefully at each of them. My opinion, previously inexperienced and untutored, matured into a carefully studied critique: now I *know* it's ridiculous. Especially for an artist who demonstrated his considerable conventional talents in his earlier work: why did he leave the Via Roma for a back alley?

But I've learned to be reverently quiet. So when they throw in elaborate orchestration and fancy cadenzas, without a genuine theme underneath all that variation, I hum *Air on the G String* or *Scheherazade* to myself. When the latest continental dish is proudly trundled out, instead of asking "Didn't you have enough for everybody? " or even "Where's the beef?" (preferably pot roast), I just eat the grilled mahi-mahi and leave the vegetables in case they want to cook them later. And when the new red rectangle is displayed on the wall of the museum, with the yellow and aquamarine splotches of acrylic, apparently flung from a distance of 12 paces, I excuse myself and repair to the Dutch Masters section, where they could at least draw.

Even Mendelssohn, however, proves to be hopeless. You can't half-listen to this kind of thing. Felix, as

255

well as Wolfgang (his dad, old Leopold, called him Wolfgang, you see, not Amadeus) and Johann Sebastian (especially Johann Sebastian) require all your concentration. Otherwise it's just noise, distraction. It takes you off the mark.

And right now I don't want to be distracted, I want to focus my full attention on sweating.

Over Randolph. If he's got a high potassium to account for his problems, it will slow and partially paralyze his heart, lowering his blood pressure. It might have caused pulmonary edema, or wet lungs. The calcium will oppose the effect of potassium on the heart. The glucose and insulin we're giving will drive the mineral into the cells, lowering the level in the blood.

Good.

The soda bicarb will correct acidosis, again causing the potassium to move out of the blood into a location inside rather than outside the cells. The heart should work better, the blood pressure should go up, the weak skeletal muscles (maybe even weak enough to impair respiration) should get stronger.

Also good.

But the sodium load may make his lungs even wetter.

Bad.

The Kayelalate will bind potassium in the intestinal tract and the Sorbitol will flush it through. Good again. But sodium will be the exchange ion, and more sodium will be absorbed. Bad again.

If all this doesn't work, we may have to put him on the artificial kidney as an emergency, correct everything. Maybe best of all.

If we're in time.

Meanwhile, the pager senses that I'm a helpless victim, pinned behind the wheel, and so it has taken advantage of the situation and beeped six more times. Some of these are undoubtedly repeats because I haven't called the last one back yet. You can sometimes sit at the phone, dial a call, get a busy signal (because the answering service is calling the patient to see if you've called), call another number, get put on hold waiting for the pharmacist, get three more beeps, hang up, call another number, there's no answer, get three more beeps because you haven't answered the previous three. That's when you develop the opinion that at some critical moment in the imminent future every single person in the world will suddenly and simultaneously get put on hold.

And the beeper will still be beeping.

THE REAL ER

Now, if you're a doctor, walking into the emergency room at Metro Hospital is an authentic thrill. On the ward you may be the invisible man; in the office just a fixture; at home that fellow who comes in, eats, then sleeps. But going into the ER you are *somebody*.

For here, some brilliant engineer, doubtless an amateur disciple of Nietzche, has created a device calculated

257

to propel the self-esteem of the physician to stratospheric heights.

It's the metal plate.

Now ordinary people go through the anteroom door, then the door into the triage area, then either head for the registration desk or sit in the waiting area, finally to be ushered through still another door into the ER.

But if you're a doctor -- and you're an *in* person -- you know about the little digital pad. You know to punch 2431. Then – the circular metal plate. The plate is located four feet to the right of the huge automatic doors. If you strike it just so with the heel of your hand -- ZOOM! The enormous doors fly open with a rush of pressurized air. And there you stand, right between the cardiac room and the major trauma unit. The waters have parted. The clouds have dissipated upon your arrival. All of them -- the ward secretary, the nurses, the aides, the ER doctor, the patients -- look up, knowing a truly significant event has transpired.

You have *arrived*!

Some cynics, like for example hospital administrators, might claim that this entry system was devised to permit emergency medical technologists instant access to the facility.

But, if you're a doctor, you know different. This is for *us*. This is the vestigial remnant of our pristine glory.

Thank you, engineer!

ON CALL FOR SURE

Tonight, though, the WHOOSH! has lost a lot of its charm because I have Randolph, the stroke, twelve beeps, and then I remember something else with a rush -- something dark and ominous.

Not that I wasn't properly informed about it.

I knew I was on call for my group: it was on the schedule.

I knew I was taking the calls of the other group, including Landers and his cronies, who are at various "meetings."*   That makes six doctors.

And I knew this too -- I'm on the emergency room medical call rotation -- I got the notice from the medical staff office.   Furthermore I've already "caught" one case of abdominal pain earlier today, in the person of Dan Godwick.

But actually *seeing* it there -- blue-crayoned on the call board right next to the ambulance radio-telephone at 10 p. m. -- gives it a special reality:

GEN SURG - Barton
NEUROSURG - Greystone
MEDICINE - Galen
PLASTIC - Grunyan
OPTH - South
PSYCH - Johnson
VASCULAR - Bagwell

"Meeting" is a code word in the medical profession. Does it conjure up visions of notepads, windowless rooms, droning presentations, thermos jugs of tepid water, and nods of assent (or, anyway, nods)? Oh, no--how could one concentrate in such an environment? One needs presentations held in a glass-walled auditorium overlooking very specific vistas such as the Hahnenkamm

downhill at Kitzbuhl, or the eighteenth of the Blue Course at Doral, or the
October foliage at the Greenbrier. Perhaps adequate audio-visual facilities,
like really good PA systems and Power Point projectors, simply cannot be found
locally. They are apparently rationed and obtainable only in $300 per-day units
like those at LaCosta, Snowbird, and the Cloister. Or why else would busy
professionals journey so far to hear programs which are, after all, scheduled
only in the mornings? Poor things, they have to concoct their own study
programs for the empty afternoons, such as geological explorations on the
Pike's Peak railway or botanical forays down the strategically planted fairways
of Pinehurst.

   I am thinking of these paradoxes as I look at the call board.

  So I'm "on" for Medicine -- meaning I automatically take calls to see any internal medical patient who is beyond the scope of the emergency room doctor, or who has no private physician and seems to need admission, or who is sort of unclassifiable. And, of course, there are all those patients of my six colleagues, in and out of the hospital, lying in wait for me, daring me to sit down, read the paper or go to the bathroom.

  I am, in sum, the target for tonight. And tonight the marksmen are lining up.

MINERAL DEPOSIT

  "Doctor Galen, am *I* glad to see *you*." Marcie is petite, cute, with a crooked little smile and a saucy attitude. But now with this particular salutation she takes on the characteristics of a witch of Endor.

"How's Randolph?"

"Looks a little better. But his potassium is 9."

Now, any internal medical or nephrology book will inform you that a normal potassium (abbreviated K+) is 3.9 to 5.4 milliequivalents per liter. It will tell you that 7 is dangerous, and that 8 is fatal. It stops the heart. In Randolph's case, however, he's undoubtedly gotten used to a high level over a long period and now, at 9, is not dead but only threatening to die.

"What about his pressure?"

"Up from 70 to 90 systolic. By Doppler."

"What's the tracing look like?"

"The QRS has narrowed, but if you slow that calcium drip below 150 it widens right out again."

"OK, put in two more amps and slow it down to 75. Don't want to overload him. Are the gases back?"

She turns and calls across the ER bay. "Henry, do you have those gases on 12?"

Henry, the respiratory technologist, walks up with a sheet of paper. Henry, somehow, in the midst of turmoil is immaculately turned out: his white coat is spotless, perfectly pressed, his haircut is recent. Only one small lock of blond hair is allowed to droop, carefully, casually over his forehead. The figures for the arterial blood gases he has inscribed in the little boxes are candidates for a calligraphy prize:

pH   7.21   PaCO2 46   paO2 59

"Was he on O2 when you drew these, Henry?"

261

"Right here, Dr. Galen." He points to a little box I had overlooked which indicates "FiO2 40%."

"Let's see, Henry, 40% really means he was on nasal O2 at what, 3 liters."

"Right."

"I guess we can afford to bump him up to 5. But that pCO2 scares me. Don't want to depress his respiration and end up with CO2 narcosis."

"True. He'd be hard to intubate, and at 300 pounds we'd have to roll in the biggest ventilator we've got."

The blood gases are instantaneously read by a machine from blood which is obtained from an artery -- in this case the radial artery in Randolph's wrist. The paO2 is the partial pressure of oxygen expressed in millimeters of mercury. Normally above 80, in Randolph's case it's only 59 even with oxygen flowing into his nose. Below 55 becomes critical. The pCO2, when someone is gasping for breath, usually goes down, indicating increased respiratory effort. Here, although Randolph is short of breath, his pCO2 is not low but slightly high. His breathing muscles aren't doing the job. And the pH, indicating acidity or alkalinity, should be 7.35-7.45, so Randolph is acidotic -- partly from the kidney failure, maybe partly from his poor breathing.

"Why do you think he's hypoventilating, Dr. Galen? Does he have lung disease?"

"No, Henry. I think it's from the high K+ -- hyperkalemic neuromyopathy." I roll this one off my tongue, so as to make Henry more respectful.

We walk into the Cardiac Room, which is called Number 12.   This chamber is across the aisle from the Trauma Room, which is called number 1.   Cardiac, 12; Trauma, 1.   Clearly, the surgeons are in charge of the ER.

"Randolph, they get you off a deer stand for this?"

His smile is as big as his massive extended hand. "Shore wish I was on a stand right now.   I don't feel that hot, doctor."

His wife, Joanne, is sitting beside the stretcher looking pale, shaking her head.   Unlike Randolph she is petite, with small ankles and wrists.   She is blonde and is wearing a flowered print dress.

"Joanne, you okay?"

"Not really, Dr. Galen, with him this way."

Using the regular blood pressure cuff, I get 60 millimeters of mercury systolic.   The Doppler, a more sensitive device which "hears" better than humans, says 85. Pulse is about 50 per minute -- slow.   His lungs sound clear, but he seems in respiratory distress, even though the oxygen is going in through a little tusk in his nose.   His neck veins are full with his head elevated at about 45 degrees.

"You pretty short of breath, Randolph?"

"Short of everything, Doctor.   Yessir, can't seem to get enough air in."

Randolph's EKGs are alarming.   A normal tracing, I know, should look something like this:

R

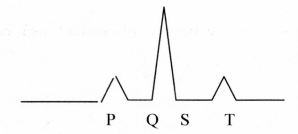

P   Q   S   T

(The labeling of points on the EKG -- P,Q,R,S,T,U -- is not the result of some recondite knowledge. Somebody just used the alphabet.)

Rapidly, I do a mental review of the changes produced by too much potassium. The earliest elevations -- at a level of 6 to 7 -- usually cause the T wave to get peaked:

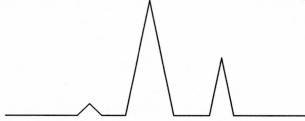

When the K+ rises into the 7-8 range, the QRS normally widens, thus:

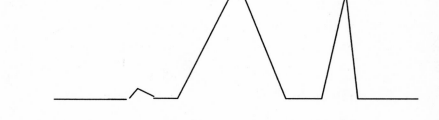

About this time, or over 8, the P waves flatten and disappear, and the heart rate slows.

Then a "sine wave," an ineffective electrical discharge, develops. At this point the heart isn't working.

264

This is the equivalent of ventricular fibrillation: that is, cardiac arrest is here.

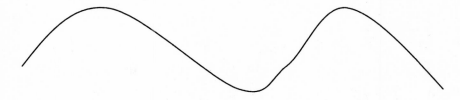

In Randolph's case, we have:

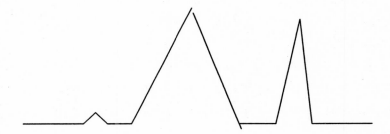

And then after our early treatment:

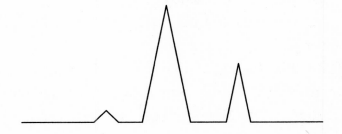

But now he's slipping back:

265

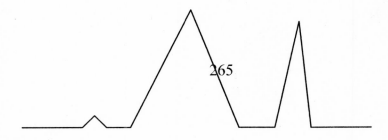

"Two more amps of bicarb, Marcie. Another calcium. Push them both. Don't we have the rest of the chemistries?"

"Here." Marcie hands me a printout. The dot-matrix printer needs a new ribbon, but it's legible:

Na 136 K 9.0 (checked) CO2 12 Cl 98   BUN 112   Creat 12.6

K+ very high; CO2, or bicarbonate level, quite low, indicating acidosis, a feature of kidney disease.   High creatinine and BUN -- "poisons" which build up in kidney failure.

"What about the film, Marcie?"

"There." She points to the fluorescent viewbox set into the wall, where the chest x-ray hangs.

"Heart's enlarged," I observe. "Moderate amount of pulmonary congestion."

"Think this is going to do it?" Marcie says.

I stare at her through slitted lids and walk into the hall. She recognizes the signal: *Come outside.*

"No," I say to Marcie, still staring. "This is not going to do it. Call the hemodialysis nurse. Let me speak to her."

BEEPER

266

I walk out to the main nursing station desk, bend over the counter, and hold up the beeper, which even now continues its jungle rhythm.

"Ginger."

The twenty-something unit secretary has blue eyes and brown hair, the random waves of which are matted down as if she's just finished a swim and hasn't had time to dry it yet. There are innumerable individual spikes trailing over her forehead. She has on an unpressed, deconstructed Madras blouse and a pair of off-white cotton cargo or carpenter's pants with about 12 pockets. Her shoes are by Nike and look appropriate for a moderately technical mountain climb. She seems, in the main, ready for a beach party where you build a bonfire and cook crabs and lobsters. In other words, in October in this strange time and this modern city she is right in style.

But she has apparently had an upbringing which was medieval, or else thinks I am, for she uses an anachronism:

"Yes, sir."

"This thing is full of messages." I hand it to her. "Could you call the answering service and see if any are urgent? I'm swimming around in patients here."

"Yes, sir, I will, and I hate to tell you this."

"What did you say, Ginger?"

"I said I really hate to tell you this --"

"Tell me."

"They have two more for you in the back."

STROKE

Minnie Jones peers at me pensively as I approach her stretcher in Room 3. She smiles faintly. I notice that the right side of her face smiles more than the left.

Good. Probably a non-dominant lesion.

Minnie, according to the demographic sheet prepared in ER admissions, is a 58-year-old black hypertensive diabetic patient of Dr. Williams, my partner. Seated in the chair beside the stretcher is a middle-aged woman who could be her sister. According to the ER sheet, she is. She happens to be dressed to the nines: silk dress, hat, pearls. She is the first to speak.

"The neighbors and that there visiting nurse said not to bother to bring her, doctor. Said it's just a stroke, and you cain't do nothing for that. But I knowed from the papers that they're using medicines and sometimes operating on veins nowadays."

She looks at the floor and shakes her head. "And it's funny, you know. It keeps coming and going. Her arm and leg gets weak, then they're all right. Then they gets weak again. And her face will be crooked when she smiles, and then it's straight again. I thought the doctor should say."

"You were very wise." *Brilliant is more like it: without the educational background you've given a classic description of the waxing and waning phenomenon of transient cerebral ischemic attack and appreciated its significance; can you, by any chance, arrange to lecture to the medical students next week?* "Mrs. -- Andrews, is it?" I'm looking at the sheet again.

"Yes. Josephine Andrews. I'm her sister."

"Dr. Galen, Dr. Williams' partner." I shake hands with Mrs. Andrews and then with Mrs. Jones. Her right handgrip is firm.

"How's your speech, Mrs. Jones?"

"Oh, fine, Doctor." She turns her head toward me with eyes closed. "And Dr. Williams just calls me Minnie." Then she pops her eyes open and smiles broadly. The smile is already a little less crooked.

"Minnie, are you right-handed or left-handed?"

"Right. Well, sometimes I eats with my left hand. But I writes with my right."

"Can you swallow all right now?"

"Yessir."

"Headache?"

"No, sir.

"Any injuries? Have you hit your head any time lately, Minnie?"

"No, sir."

"Exactly how did this come on?"

"Just weakness, Doctor. I cain't hold nothing in my left hand. And my left leg won't hold me. And then like Josephine says they both gets all right. Been doing this all afternoon."

Her blood pressure is 180/110, pulse 72. The facial lag has now completely gone. The strength in her arms and legs seems intact. Detailed neurological examination now shows only two rather subtle residues of her affliction: drift and the Babinski sign.

Drift shows up when Minnie holds both arms straight ahead with her eyes closed. The right holds its position, demonstrating the incredible capacity of the nervous system to integrate floods of proprioceptive impulses and respond with showers of tiny directions to the muscles of posture -- a routine miracle. But the left sags rhythmically downward, like a conductor leading a ritard -- andante, then adagio.

I stroke the outside of the soles of Minnie's feet, first right, then left. The right response is normal: the toes curl downward slightly. But on the left, they extend, spread, and the big toe rocks upward. This minor difference, first noted by Dr. Babinski, was a revolutionary finding in his time -- as crucial to progress as the MRI scanner is today. I know that this sign, usually referred to by the medical cognoscenti as the extensor plantar response, means there is trouble between the cerebral cortex and the point where the nerve to the foot exits from the spinal cord. Normally the higher brain centers exert an inhibiting effect; now this braking influence is impaired and the primitive extension of the toes, normal in young infants, returns. Minnie's left foot has regressed to infancy, to ancient animal forms. Like the newborn, her foot has now been freed from the sophisticated evolutionary bonds of the human neocortex and, here in the emergency room, happily splays. But, we hope, temporarily.

The carotid arteries, examined carefully with the stethoscope, show no significant bruit: the rhythmic roar of a blocked vessel is absent. These big conduits of blood to Minnie's brain are not exonerated by this silence, but at least their guilt is not obvious.

270

Since cerebral control of the body is crossed, I know that it is the right side of Minnie's brain which is affected and which results in her intermittent left-sided weakness. The control of speech is lodged in the dominant hemisphere, which is virtually always on the left in right-handed people (in left-handed people this is variable). Meanwhile, that strange right side is given credit for more and more things these days -- creativity, insight, intuition. Maybe so. Certainly much reflex behavior lodges there: the perfect pirouette, the flawless ski turn, the effortless golf swing. But it's strange -- people who have strokes in this right side sometimes show bizarre behavior: they become inattentive; they develop an automatic, often hilarious, sense of humor. In any event Minnie's right-sided brain, left-sided body stroke is leaving her speech unaffected even during the periods when the weakness episodically returns. Lucky for Minnie.

But somewhere in that faltering right hemisphere, a blood vessel is failing. It is probably threatening to close down. A clot may be forming, or tiny clots may be breaking off upstream and causing these spells. If the clot blocks the vessel completely, damage to brain tissue -- an infarction -- may occur. Anticoagulants at this stage may help.

But in medicine, I've learned, things are often not what they seem, and the books don't always cover it. A small artery could have ruptured, after all. An area of bleeding could have developed. The size of the blood collection could be waxing and waning, producing the changeable signs Minnie is showing. Then anticoagulants could be disastrous.

We need to tell the difference, if we can, and fast.

271

Marcie dashes in, her hands full of IV tubing and tape. "Eight-point- two now, Dr. Galen."

"What?"

"The K+. Eight-point-two. On Randolph. You with me?"

"That's good, or at least a little better. I was consulting with Dr. Babinski."

"Who?"

"Nothing. Let's get a head CT on Minnie here. Without contrast. Stat. And get her a room."

"You got it . . . . without contrast." She turns and signals to Ginger. "Uh, Dr. Galen--"

"Yes?"

"Dr. Babinski?"

"Yes."

"Is he on our staff?"

"No."

STOMACH TROUBLE

I plot a course to check on Randolph and then see an advertised "strep throat," but Ginger intercepts me.

"What admission diagnosis on Jones, in 3, Doctor Galen?"

"TIA."

"That's transient ischemic attack?"

"Yeah. Attacks. And I'm going to 12 and then 8."

"Well, Dr. Galen, two of these calls are pretty urgent, or the patients say they are. Number 6 and number 13 on the pager." She holds up the instrument, which resembles a grey cigarette package.

CALL 6 - 9:56 - 636-9662 - MRS DEMOREST - NAUSEA AND VOMITING

"Hello." The female voice is subdued, somewhat hoarse.

"Mrs. Demorest, I hear you're having some trouble."

"Vomiting since about four o'clock, Doctor. Can't keep anything down, even water."

"Any abdominal pain?"

"No."

"Diarrhea?"

"Not yet."

"Fever?"

"I haven't taken it. I don't think so. Maybe I'm a little chilly."

"Anyone in the family sick?"

"No. Just me."

"Any unusual food in the last twenty-four hours?"

"No. Well, shrimp last night at a seafood restaurant. But my husband and daughter ate there too and they're OK."

"All right. Take nothing by mouth for a few hours. I'm going to send you some Phenergan suppositories. Use them every four hours. If this doesn't settle down by morning so you can take liquids, call me back. Or report any new symptoms anyway."

"Thank you, Doctor. My regular druggist is closed, but there's a National open down the street. 633-8864."

CALL 13 - 10:12 - 233-9889 - RICHARD EGBERT - WIFE HAS ABDOMINAL PAIN.

"What's the pain like, Mr. Egbert?"
"Well, I think it's in her stomach area."
"May I speak to her?"
"She doesn't feel like coming to the phone, Doctor."
"Can you ask her exactly where the pain is?"
"Just a minute."
Pause.
"She says it's down on the right side."
"When did it come on?"
"Just a minute."
Pause.
"About one o'clock this afternoon."
"Has she had her appendix out?"
"What?"
"Has she had her appendix--"
"Just a minute."
Pause.
"No."
"Mr. Egbert, I know you wife is feeling ill and doesn't want to come to the phone, but I'm afraid we'll have to examine her. Can you bring her to the emergency clinic? Can she ride in a car?"
"Just a minute."

Pause.

"She says she can."

In Room 12 Randolph somehow looks a little better. The curly graying hair and prominent sideburns form a halo around his already huge head, making it seem larger still. His color is still pallid. His blood pressure, ordinarily 140/80, is still 90 by Doppler. His lungs still show rales. The neck veins are still strutted. But some of the desperation has gone from his face.

Marcie has turned the case over to Charles, a tall, efficient but laconic male nurse.

"Charles, we'd better get another K+, the third one."

"Yessir, actually I went ahead and sent one."

I turn to Randolph. "Looking better, big man. How're you feeling?"

"Better, Doc. But nothin' extra."

Ginger appears at the door. "Gloria from dialysis on 3298." She holds up a telephone with about a 40-foot cord.

"Hear the K+s are running high tonight," Gloria says.

"What? You mean the lab's having a problem?"

"No -- no. I meant Randolph. They said his was 9."

"Yeah, right. I doubt we'll be able to handle it or the fluid volume without emergency hemo."

"I'm up here in inpatient setting up right now. Will he go to ICU?"

"Yes."

"OK, I'll do him there."

"Great. Zero K+ bath. And we'll need to diafiltrate."

275

"Right. See you in a little while. Who's going to put in an access?"

"I put in a call to Bagwell. He's on ER call, anyway. Probably put in a subclavian, a Quinton or something. Any problem with that we'll stick in femoral caths."

"Good."

Randolph looks thoughtful. "Guess I'm gonna have to go for that transplant pretty soon, eh, Doc?"

"I guess so, Randolph. They've already activated you since your workup on the unit, you know."

"Yeah, they sent me a letter and a beeper."

"But you know, Randolph, now we may have to start dialysis on a regular basis before then."

"Yeah, you been threatening that."

Now it's Charles who hands me the telephone with the long cord. "Dr. Bagwell for you."

"Stanley, thanks for calling back."

"Sure."

"Looks like we've got an emergency dialysis problem here. Came in with a K+ of 9. Overloaded. We're making only slow progress. Just a second, please."

Charles holds up the newest strip. It looks like the T waves are getting sharper again, the QRS is narrower, the pulse is slower.

"EKG keeps reverting to a bad hyperkalemic picture. Can you put in a subclavian?"

"No problem. Where are you?"

"ER, number 12, but headed for ICU -- which ICU, Charles?"

"ICU-Green."

"Green, Stanley. We'll dialyze him there. Name's Randolph Brown."

"Be there in ten minutes. Can I speak to the dialysis nurse?"

"She's in the inpatient unit -- 3529."

"Right. I'll call her to get the stuff."

"Thanks – a whole lot."

STREP

"Ginger, how're you doing now?"

She covers the mouthpiece of the telephone. "OK if I can just get the lab to answer. What about you?"

"Moving right along. Room 8 next."

The sheet says that Doug Hutton is a 34-year-old computer programmer who thinks he has a strep throat. I sigh. Another one. You see, 80 percent of sore throats are not due to the streptococcus. In fact, they aren't bacterial at all, they're viral. If so, there's no specific treatment -- just relieve pain, use a gargle, decide if antibiotics are needed to prevent secondary infection (this is debatable). So here's Doug, reporting in with a sore throat at 10:30 p.m. Has probably had it for three days, didn't bother to call Dr. Lehigh.

But the fact is, Doug has stumbled tonight upon a doctor who has deep respect for strep throats. . . because I had one in the pre-antibiotic era. In fact, in the pre-sulfa era. At age eight I was in bed at home for three weeks. I was delirious most nights. There was a general surgeon who came occasionally, an ENT doctor who came periodically, the pediatrician who came daily, and my physician-father who checked on me three times a day. I had (embarrassing) private-duty nurses around the clock. My mother was on permanent duty. One day the surgeon came, examined me, and said it had drained, he didn't have to incise the abscess after all. I remember I was happy to hear that and happy I had never known enough to worry about it in the first place. There were many unpleasant memories of my strep throat, but the worst was the enema. You see, if I didn't perform for 48 hours, I got the enema. I watched the clock tick toward enema time; sometimes they forgot and I went over schedule, but I made sure it was never early.

Later, after a full recovery, I was glad the abscess had drained spontaneously, glad the bad dreams were over. I was happy there were no more embarrassing private-duty nurses. I was even glad to get back to school. But the thing I was most glad about was: no more enemas.

In retrospect, what I should have really been delighted over was not having the late complications of streptococcal infection: rheumatic fever, which affects the heart, or glomerulonephritis, which affects the kidneys. The streptococcal germ shows up on a Gram-stained slide as little round purple balls lined up in chains. Some of the subspecies and strains of this innocent-looking bug have the property of altering the protein of heart tissue so that the body mistakenly makes antibodies against its own flesh. The heart becomes inflamed, the muscle flags, the chambers dilate, the organ fails to perform its appointed task of pumping. Acute rheumatic myocarditis is rare now, but it was a fearsome thing: the lungs of the patient, usually a child, become engorged with fluid. Shortness of breath, even death could result. If the little patient survives, he or she may later suffer the effects of valvular deformity -- narrowing, or just as bad, leakage -- of the mitral or aortic openings.

A similar type of thing can happen to the kidneys. Apparently some complex of the streptococcus and antibody finds its way to the little vascular tufts, called glomeruli. This antigen-antibody complex, like so much gunk, plugs up the tiny glomerular capillaries. An inflammatory reaction sets in, damage to the filtering unit occurs, and scarring takes place. The kidney leaks protein into the urine, swelling of the body occurs, and eventually, kidney failure supervenes. With antibiotics, the process can sometimes be aborted. Rheumatic fever is getting to be an oddity, mostly seen in the New England states. Acute glomerulonephritis is on the wane, too, although a related, less-well-understood, chronic process is still the most common cause for renal insufficiency in young people. I remember that Karen was thought to have both rheumatic fever and glomerulonephritis at the same time – until we diagnosed lupus.

In any event, nowadays, a strep throat responds within 48 hours to penicillin or one of its many relatives. Even erythromycin is effective. Sore throat, fever -- zap! -- you're well.

But penicillin or not, viral preponderance or not, it is with reverent respect that I approach Doug.

"Hi, doctor," he says.

And from the way he says it, I know. This time the preliminary billing is probably correct: Jim does indeed have a strep throat. He keeps his mouth open. His consonants are slurred. His voice is a monotone. He has, in short, a diffuse swelling of his pharyngeal tissues due to the cellulitis which the streptococcus characteristically produces. It changes the voice. Swallowing is difficult. Pediatricians boast they can diagnose it over the telephone.

Examination confirms the suspicion. His throat is carmine-red -- indeed, a sibling of this strep is the one which produces the toxin of scarlet fever. Doug, then, can be said to have scarlet throat. The tissues are bulging, glistening. The tonsils are hugely enlarged. There is a patchy white exudate over the tonsillar fauces and the posterior pharynx. Under the angles of his jaws are large tender masses of reactive cervical lymph nodes, often called "glands" -- the "tonsillar nodes." His temperature, taken earlier by the nurse with an electronic probe inserted for seconds into the external ear canal, is recorded at 101.6 degrees F (38.9 C).

"What about it, Dr. Galen?" Marcie, the ever-present monitor.

"Strep. But of course there's one possible hooker -- mono. Let's get a white count with diff, a mono spot, a rapid strep screen, and a culture. But I've seen enough. We'll treat."

"OK," says Marcie.

"Good," says Doug.

"It says here you're allergic to penicillin, Doug."

"Yessir, well, I'm not positive. I think I had a rash after a shot when I was a child."

"The blood tests will be back in a few minutes. Then we'll go ahead and start you on medication while we're waiting for the results of the culture -- that'll be 24-48 hours. We'll give you one of the multi-purpose cousins of penicillin, but the chance of a cross-reaction is very small."

"Whatever, Doc," he says in his monotone.

The drug I select is cephalexin, a time-tested first-generation member of the cephalosporin group. This family provides a wonderful array of antibacterial agents with powerful activity against a broad spectrum of offending bugs. There are now five generations of these drugs with about five to eight in each category. Only the infectious disease specialists can keep them all straight: ordinary MDs pick a single favorite in each generation and go about their business.

The screen is positive. So Doug knows he has a strep throat. He knows he'll get an antibiotic and get well in a day or two.

But I know some other things. Doug, you won't be sick in bed three weeks. You won't be delirious. You won't have private-duty nurses, worried parents, an abscess, glom-erulonephritis, or rheumatic fever.

And, Doug -- you won't get any enemas.

Marcie hands me a fragment of paper. It is Randolph's latest tracing. "Strip looks worse."

"Is this a precordial lead?"

"Yep."

281

"Same lead as before? It looks like a different one."

"I'll check."

"Seen Bagwell?"

"He's in there now. Putting in the line. Having trouble because Randolph's so big and short-necked."

"OK, better see about that tracing."

ROUTINE Rx

I flip open my cell phone. The beeper says:

IDLEWOOD PHARMACY PHONE BOOTH - 994-3976 - WANDA EDWARDS.

In fact, it says that three times, at 9:58, 10:24, and now, at 10:46.

I don't know Wanda.

She says: "My father just died and I've got to go to Indianapolis on the 3 o'clock plane. My migraine is flaring up. My regular doctor is Dr. -- Blank. He usually gives me Tylenol Number 3, 30 of them. I'll see Dr. -- Blank when I get back. Will you talk to the druggist? His number back here is 404-237-5492."

"Sure, Wanda, I'll talk to him."

"Right. Thanks, Doctor."

I dial the number and the telephone buzzes.

"Pharmacist."

"Dr. John Galen. Are you aware of Wanda Edwards there in your store?"

"Oh, Dr. Galen. Jim Moore here. There *is* a girl up there using the pay phone. Looks a little familiar."

"She's calling trying to get Tylenol with codeine. Sounded like she was reading from a prepared form. Said her doctor was Dr. *Blank,* for God's sake."

"Really? We're seeing more of that type of thing, but they're hard to prosecute. I'll call the police but they may not even come for a little codeine. Give me the name again. And the prescription."

"Wanda Edwards. Tylenol Number 3, number 30. But don't fill it, of course."

"'Course not. I'll fiddle around hoping the police will get here. *Dr. Blank,* eh?"

"Yes. I'll call you later to find out what happened. How late are you open?"

"Twelve. Thanks, Doctor Galen."

"Thank you, Dr. Moore."

Marcie again. "Woman back in 6, you know, Dr. Galen. Patient of Dr. Fitzgibbon's. Man with her keeps agitating. Says her face is paralyzed, says she's had a stroke. Been waiting about an hour."

"Thanks, Marcie. I know. Sorry. Serve them some tea."

"What?"

"Where do we stand with Randolph?"

"Here's the new tracing. Went ahead and did a 12-lead. Not much change from before. I think you were right

283

about the other lead. The electrode was in a funny precordial position."

The newest tracing shows a better picture, much like the one which had improved with treatment.

"Marcie, this just goes to show you. With EKGs as with fruit, one must separate the apples from the persimmons. Lead 1 is not Lead 2 is not Lead 3, and those strips which come out of the monitor shall not dominate the earth."

"Dr. Galen, I know you're *on* tonight. But are you *on anything*?"

"Just the milk of human kindness, Marcie."

"Whatever you say. Anyway, ICU Green is ready for Randolph. In fact, they're moving him now. The catheter is in. A Uldall, I think."

WET READING

"Heard anything about Minnie Jones' CT scan?"

"I think Ginger's got a wet reading. GINGER!"

Ginger raises her hand with a piece of paper in it, waving, and runs over to where we're standing in the aisle. *Wet reading* is an honored medical anachronism. The term comes from the time when all X-rays were hand-developed. You would put the film, clamped in its metal frame, into the developer for 6 minutes, then rinse for 3 minutes, then put it in the fixer for 10 minutes, then rinse again. Then you would hold it up to the viewbox and try to interpret it. Strange and wonderful things could happen to the film as it dried, so that interesting mistakes could be made. Thus *wet reading* was the quintessential disclaimer: "It appears that so-and-so is

284

present, but of course this must be confirmed with a dry reading." Now X-rays are dry and ready within a couple of minutes. Indeed, the computer projects them on the radiologist's telemonitor in real time.

"You're well named, Ginger."

"That's what my mother says."

The emergency report is concise. It says: *Minnie Jones Pt. #00075603   ER 10:37 PM 10/22.   Head CT scan. Minimal atrophy.   No lesions.   No evidence of hemorrhage. John Wilkerson, MD.*

Now John is a highly trained radiologist. But he is not sitting here tonight in a windowless room (we internists call it Valley of the Shadows). He is at home, availing himself of the wonderful new technology which permits the digital pictures from the CT scan to be projected on a screen, perhaps on his bedside table. My partner Elbert says the radiologists have "radial nerve palsy," an affliction which results from compressing the nerve when one leans on one's arm to look at a screen without getting up out of bed. We hear some hospitals beam nighttime images to India, so that radiologists there can read the X-rays during daylight hours. In any event, thanks to technology and John, we have a final and expert opinion on Minnie's brain. In a moment I can look at the screen myself (and pretend to be an expert).

"Minnie still down here, Ginger?"

"Yes. Number Three. Lisa's taking care of her now. *Lisa!*"

Lisa looks up from the computer at the long desk. "Is that the CT report?"

"Yeah," I say. "Negative. No hemorrhage. Too early to know if an infarction is developing. That may take a few days to show up. Anyway, it's safe to anticoagulate her. Let's give a her a loading dose of heparin. 4,000 units IV push, then hang a drip, 700 units an hour, in D-5-W. First get labs-- the usual CBC, SMA-6. Also a PT, PTT. I'll write the orders in a minute. Get out a copy of the heparin protocol. I've got to serve some tea."

"You listening, Lisa?" asks Ginger. "I can't take orders, you know, Dr. Galen, I'm not an RN."

"I know."

"I'm listening, I'm listening." Lisa is scribbling. "Right. Let me read it back. CBC, SMA-6, PT, PTT stat. Then aqueous heparin 4000 units IV stat, then 700 units an hour in D-5-W. You'll fill out the protocol. You've got to go do *what*?"

"I've got to go to Room 6."

NON-STROKE

Louise Whitmore is a 36-year-old interior designer sitting on a stool in Room 6. She is trim, attractive, has brown hair, unexpectedly blue eyes, and is flawlessly groomed. But now she looks distraught.

Or she would if the right side of her face could move. The left half is mobile, smiling, then frowning. The right droops, expressionless. The forehead wrinkles are ironed out

286

on that side.   The angle of the mouth is drawn downward. She reminds me of Minnie Jones but with a big difference.

Her companion -- he is identified only as Significant Other by the unintended irony of the computer form -- doesn't look distraught, he looks irritated.   He has on a solid gray suit with a puff handkerchief in the pocket.   His hair is long, prematurely white, wavy, and has a coiffed look.

"Dr. John Galen, Ms. Whitmore."   I shake hands with her and then turn to her companion.

"Anderson Forsyth," he says.   "Glad to see you finally.   We've had to wait quite a while."

"Yes, I know.   Sorry.   A bunch of emergencies here."

"Oh, *really?*   Well, what about *this* emergency? Doesn't a stroke qualify?   Or do you have to get an affidavit?"

I'm looking at Ms. Whitmore, not Forsyth.   "Happy to say this doesn't look like a stroke.   And, fortunately, I'm even more delighted to say I believe we don't have an emergency here."

"How do you know? Nobody's even examined her."

Sylvia Whitmore speaks: "If you'll be quiet, Andy, maybe he can."

I smile tolerantly and start to do another neurological examination.   Twenty years ago I might well have gotten angry at Forsyth's display; now I recognize it as just that – an act.   Forsyth (not I) has something to prove, perhaps to Ms. Whitmore.   *I am macho after all,* he may well be saying. *The times you've thought I caved in on important issues didn't mean anything.   Here is my dominant male personality asserting itself.   I'm the one who insisted you come in and get*

287

this checked instead of going to the play and I was the one who said I'd get you immediate attention -- and here I am, foiled by the system. I'll show them -- and you, my dear.

You see, *I* don't have a problem, Mr. Forsyth has the problem. I'm just plugging along, doing my best. He's the one on stage. This is not bothering me at all. Much. I think. However, I go ahead anyway and decide to use one of the physician's most powerful time-honored weapons.

"Mr. Forsyth, if you'll excuse us for a few minutes, I'll finish examining Ms. Whitmore."

"Go ahead."

"I mean, would you mind stepping out for a moment?"

"I don't believe that will be necessary."

Ms. Whitmore's eyes and her right index finger are not paralyzed. They all three fix on Forsyth. "Anderson, go out in the hall."

He looks at Louise, then me, then the wall. Then he leaves the room.

Unlike Minnie Jones, Louise has no weakness anywhere except for the face. There is no drift. No loss of sensation, even in the paralyzed area. No Babinski. And most critical of all, her facial weakness involves not just the lower part but the eye and forehead as well. In attempting to raise her eyebrows, only the left goes up. In closing her eyes, only the left eyelid closes. The right gapes pathetically and the right eye, as if seeking cover, rolls upward. The entire right face is flat, free of crow's feet, devoid of tone. She has undergone a Botox-like experiment of nature.

Minnie has a central facial weakness; Louise has a peripheral facial paralysis. Minnie has a threatened stroke; Louise, a virus.

I open the door and, without looking out, say, "You can come back in, Mr. Forsyth."

He walks in, arms folded across his chest.

"This is Bell's palsy," I say to Louise, with more calm confidence than is perhaps warranted.

"And what the hell is that?" asks Forsyth.

I am so impervious that I ignore him. "When did this actually come on, Ms. Whitmore?"

"This afternoon. I took a nap after an appointment and when I woke up it was there. Just can't move the right side of my face at all."

"Any pain?"

"No, just a funny feeling on the right side. Kind of numb, but I can really feel normally."

"When will she recover?" Forsyth is still standing now, arms still clutching his torso.

Still emotionally uninvolved, I nonetheless decide to continue his punishment. "Ms. Whitmore, have you had any colds, or sore throats, or fever lately?"

"Well, I have had a little sniffles for the last couple of days. Felt a little bit chilly last night."

Now I turn to Forsyth, rather majestically, I think, and then to the wall between them, as if addressing a class. I take off my glasses. I've seen professors take off their glasses when they are about to deliver critical messages.

289

"Bell's palsy is an acute disorder of the seventh, or facial nerve," I begin. "This is the motor nerve to the face, and so the face becomes paralyzed on that side."

Forsyth is stony-faced. "Isn't palsy a tremor?"

"Palsy means paralysis," I continue, with just the faintest glimmer of a tolerant smile. "And here there is no loss of sensation. You may notice that the entire right face is paralyzed. In a stroke, only the lower part of the face is ordinarily affected. The forehead works normally. The eyelid closes normally. Here the whole side is paralyzed. The nerve isn't working. Now--"

"What brings it on?" Forsyth is still directing the interrogation.

"Now --" I go on, "the cause of Bell's palsy has never been conclusively identified. Most authorities believe it can be caused by a number of neurotropic viruses. There is about an 80-per-cent chance of complete recovery without treatment --"

"Well, of course we want Louise to have specific treatment --"

"-- And unfortunately there is no specific treatment. Currently it is thought that early use of corticosteroids will increase the chance of recovery substantially, and so I would recommend --"

"When are we going to see a neurologist and have a CAT scan?" Forsyth still.

I am so cool I amaze myself. "I don't think that's necessary, but if Ms. Whitmore wishes, I'll be happy to arrange consultation --"

290

She speaks up, her articulation slightly impaired by the sagging mouth. "No, doctor, I don't want to see anyone else unless you think I need to."

Forsyth keeps going. "Well, surely you're going to do a CAT scan at least, or preferably an MRI."

"I don't believe it will show us anything at all."

"How do you know it's not a tumor?" Forsyth continues.

"Tumors don't behave this way. They generally show slow progression, not a sudden onset. Also, it would be almost unheard-of for a tumor to involve only one peripheral nerve and not cause any other neurological findings. It would, frankly, be rather unorthodox to do a scan on a patient with Bell's --"

"But if we were in a court of law, you couldn't prove she doesn't have a tumor, now could you?"

"No."

"That's what I thought."

"I couldn't prove *you* don't have one."

"What?"

"Do you want a CAT scan?"

"Don't be absurd. I'm not part of this contract."

"Forsyth, are you by any chance either a physician or a lawyer?"

"No, of course not. An architect, why?"

"That's a relief. Then all this medical and legal advice is free."

291

Louise breaks in. "Anderson, go outside and get the car started. Turn on the heater. I'll be out in a minute. I want to talk to the doctor. I'll talk to you later."

Forsyth doesn't move. "Well, I just want to say that I think this whole thing is pretty helter-skelter. Patient comes into an emergency facility, waits an hour, doctor tries to cover up by saying that everybody knew she didn't have a stroke or anything serious. Now that would be hard to document, wouldn't it? Then, no effort made to prove what she has or doesn't have. No scans, no consultations, no labwork at all. Everything sort of off-hand."

"Sorry you feel that way, Forsyth. In my opinion the history and examination is all that's necessary to document this diagnosis. A neurologic consultant would agree. And he'd charge about $150 -- that's a lot more than I will. He undoubtedly wouldn't want a CT scan or MRI -- that'll save eight hundred dollars. Labwork would all be normal and would be down the drain. That's another hundred. It takes a little training and experience to know what to do and sometimes a lot more to know what *not* to do. But in this case it doesn't really take much."

"Exactly what do you mean by that?"

"Look at this nursing evaluation." I hold up the clipboard. In the block labeled "Comment" the note says "Complete peripheral-type facial paralysis compatible with neuritis of the seventh nerve. Jessica Tate, RN."

"She's just guessing."

"Good guess. And this, Forsyth." I have dropped the mister. I flip back several sheets to a note by Jim, the admission clerk. Jim is a high-school graduate, planning college soon -- quite a bright fellow.

"Patient reports paralysis of the right face. Looks like Bell's palsy."

"So even the clerk can diagnose it, huh?" Forsyth says.

"Even the clerk."

Forsyth walks out the door.

"I'm sorry for all that, Doctor," says Louise. "Sometimes he gets a little ruffled."

"No problem, Ms. Whitmore. The important thing is to get you straightened out. This condition, as I say, usually gets completely well, but that's not always true. I recommend that you take this prescription for prednisone, then gradually taper off. You need to be followed weekly by Dr. Frankman. You may need some physical therapy later. Right now you need to use an eyepatch, especially at night, to protect your cornea. And I would put this other prescription in your eye four times a day to prevent drying. You haven't had a stroke, and you don't have a tumor, just neuritis of the facial nerve. Questions?"

"I guess not. Any special diet?"

"No."

"Limitation on activities?"

"No."

"Is alcohol OK?"

"Yes, in moderation."

"Should I avoid sex?"

Now I'm really being tested. I can feel Mephistopheles crawling up my back. He has his talons in my spine. He is, after all this time, still tingling over his encounter with Faust, glowing with victory, the poor man's soul tucked comfortably under his red cape. He figures that I am a brother to Dr. Faustus. But I take a deep breath and shake him off.

"No, Mrs. Whitmore. No limitation."

PUTTING RANDOLPH ON

Ginger is standing hipshot in the main bay of the ER, head tilted, rueful smile on her face, with the long-cord phone in her hand. "Gloria. For you. They're getting ready to hook Randolph up."

"Thanks." I take the phone. "Gloria? How about it?"

"OK. Just want to make sure about a few things. I've got a zero-K+ bath. I'm going to try to use a 3400-C kidney, he's big and overloaded, but I'm afraid to go to a 6200 because he's hypotensive."

"Good."

"I'll plan to dump the prime, run him with as high a venous pressure as he'll take without dropping out."

"I'll buy all that. How's his pressure holding since y'all moved him?"

"About the same -- 90 systolic."

"OK. Go ahead and put him on. His pressure will undoubtedly fall out when you turn on the pump. But I wouldn't give him volume. No albumin, either. If you have to, hang a Dopamine drip, it should be temporary. His BP

294

should come up right away as soon as some of the K+ dialyzes out. I'll be there as soon as I can make a dent in the night clinic here . . .Uh-oh."

"What's the matter?"

"MVA. They're bringing in two on stretchers right now. They were supposed to go to Methodist, I heard Marcie tell them on the radio we were on bypass because of those other two trauma patients. Gloria, you'd better just go ahead and call the resource nurse for us and tell her it's hit the fan over here. Get help, any kind."

TRIAGE

When you have to juggle priorities in medicine, you call it *triage.* The rigid hierarchy of responsibility which puts Randolph, Minnie, Doug, Louise, and all those calls in my lap is not inviolable. Now with two blood-covered bodies -- products of a Motor Vehicle Accident -- being wheeled in, both on long boards with necks in rigid collars, one intubated and being bagged by an EMT, the other looking shocky, I reassess my role. I'm not an ER doc, not an ER nurse, not an employee of the hospital. I'm not one of the general surgeons, who are supposed to handle multiple trauma. But I guess I am, after all, a doctor.

I remember the scene. The freshman medical student, a young woman, in the middle of the classroom, asked the Dean, "Are we still doctors after five o'clock?"

The Dean, clever fellow, knew just what to say: "Let's ask Dr. Galen that question."

295

I, also figuring to be clever, said, "Let's ask the class. You're on the way with your Significant Other to the cocktail party. It's 6 p.m. and you're running late. A young man is lying beside the road beside his overturned motorcycle. No ambulance is there. What do you do?"

I pointed one by one to about eight students in turn. Each said, *You Have to Stop.* I polled the class. All 108 -- *Stop.* I turned to the original questioner and asked her opinion.

"You have to stop. My opinion was that we were always doctors," she said. "I just wanted to run the question up the flagpole."

She was smiling broadly.

In short, I drop everything and help. And not necessarily in the role of physician. In emergencies, the shortage is not usually of doctors, it's of functionaries -- people to get tape, to push stretchers around, to call respiratory techs, to help start IVs, to pump the Ambuc bag while somebody gets the ventilator, to roust out the X-ray tech. In a disaster area, you don't need doctors, you need bodies.

Lou Kendrick, MD, one of the ER physicians, is standing at the side of the stretcher of the man with the tube down his trachea and is giving orders. I go to the other stretcher, where Janet and two EMTs are checking vital signs and repositioning IV tubing. The patient is a young brown-haired, brown-eyed woman with a cupid-bow mouth like Bernadette Peters. She has blood all over her face, apparently

296

from a scalp wound. There are several small facial lacerations.

"I'll help out until Tom gets free. Which room are we going to?"

"We don't have any empty, Susie's trying to move somebody out," says Janet.

"How's the pressure?"

"Fifty systolic," says one of the EMTs, an obese young woman with red hair and a surprisingly beautiful face. She is wearing a uniform that looks like police garb. She retightens the blood pressure cuff about the arm. "But her pulse is only 43."

"What about extent of injuries?"

"Lacerations," says the redhead's male partner. He is young, dark, powerful-looking. "And complains of pain in the pelvic area, maybe some pelvic fractures, no obvious problems with chest or extremities. Pressure was 120 with pulse of 110 when we picked her up 10 minutes ago. Now it's way down. Her name's Billie."

The patient is grimacing. "Can't you please give me something for the pain?' she asks, her hand moving to her right hip area.

"In just a minute, Billie," I say. "I'm Dr. Galen. We'll take care of you. Got to make sure you're stable first. What's going here?" My hand touches the IV tubing.

"D-5-Ringers wide open," says the redhead.

"She had any atropine?"

"No."

I look at Janet. "Let's give her point five milligrams IV. This hypotension may be vasovagal, from the pain."

"Yeah," says the male technician. " A scalp laceration shouldn't drop her pressure like this."

"We don't see much blood, true, but they can sure bleed out from the scalp in no time. "

"Yeah, I've seen that too."

"And of course *any* amount of bleeding can occur with pelvic fractures. They can put several pints into the pelvis in minutes."

"Yessir."

"But here, this slow pulse makes me think we've got a vagal thing. We'll need another IV access."

"Your wish, our command," says Marcie, ahead of me as usual. She has suddenly appeared on the opposite side of the stretcher with IV tubing in her hand, a Cathlon set in her mouth, and a bag of IV fluids over one shoulder. With what seems to be a single continuous motion she unravels the IV tubing, plugs it into the bag, puts the bag back on her shoulder, hooks the Cathlon into the tubing, runs the fluid through, squirts a fine jet of clear liquid on the floor, places a tourniquet on the arm, finds a branch of the cephalic vein in the forearm, inserts the Cathlon, confirms the blood reflux, releases the tourniquet, turns up the flow with a rolling damper, hooks an IV stand with her foot from its position against a nearby wall, hangs the bag on the stand, tapes the IV in place with pieces of tape which were precut and sticking to her uniform, and looks up with a pixie smile.

"Showoff," I say.

The smile broadens. "Just making my nine to five."

"And don't forget five to nine," says Janet. "Pulse is up to 70. and BP systolic is 85 now. That's three minutes after the IV atropine."

"Good," I put in. "Don't we have a room?"

"Number 2 is open now, but not clean," says Marcie.

"What was in that room?"

"Just an ankle sprain."

"No hepatitis, HIV, or anything?"

"Not that we know of."

"OK, let's go now, clean up later."

Tom Vinson, the other ER MD, walks up. "What we got?" he asks.

I try to be terse, as if I do this every night. "MVA. Facial and scalp lacerations. Pelvic pain, poss. fractures. Vasovagal reaction. Apparently responding to atropine. Haven't really examined her yet. Needs blood sent to the lab, X-Rays, etc., she's going to 2. You free now?"

"Yeah, I'll take over. Thanks a lot."

"No problem. I've got some other fish in the pan over here."

"You sure have, Dr. Galen." It's Ginger. "This beeper is still going, which is not big news. But there"s a chest pain on here." She hands me the gray cigarette case.

The phone rings a long time, and while I'm waiting, I notice Anderson Forsyth walking back in from the parking lot. He meets Louise Whitmore in the open bay and takes her arm. She shakes her arm free. She says something I can't

hear. He shrugs broadly and says something else I can't hear.
As they reach the exit door, Louise says something again, and
this time I can hear the last word:

". . . ASSHOLE!"

ACUTE INDIGESTION

"Hello?" A female voice.

"Mrs. Adams?"

"Yes. Dr. Landers?"

"No, ma'am, this is Dr. John Galen, I'm taking calls
for Dr. Landers. I understand Mr. Adams is having some
chest pain?"

"Thank you, Doctor. Yes, he came home early, about
four, said he'd had some nagging indigestion in his chest
today. Said it would last for a few minutes, then go away."

"Can he speak to me?"

"Yes, but he's been having severe pain now for about
30 minutes. I wanted to call right away, but he said no, he'll
see how he felt in a while. I'll get him."

"No, never mind. We need to get him to this
emergency room right away. We'll call an ambulance.
Where do you live?"

"On Greycliff. Just two blocks from the hospital."

"Then never mind the ambulance. Can he get into the
car all right?"

"Oh, yes, I think so. But doesn't he need oxygen and
so forth?"

"Probably, but you can get him here in a fraction of the time it would take to get an ambulance there. Come right away. You understand?"

"Yes, doctor."

"Mrs. Adams --"

"Yes?"

"Give him an aspirin by mouth. And drive carefully, it's just two blocks."

"Marcie. MARCIE! OK, then Janet. I"ve got a chest pain coming in. Better put him in 12 if it's open. Vital signs, monitor, 12-lead, O2, you know, the usual. His wife is bringing him by car. Adams."

"OK, Dr. Galen. We'll call you. But a chest pain -- why no ambulance?"

"We didn't have time."

Janet looks puzzled. "Oh," she says.

"He lives two blocks away. He'll be here in five minutes. The ambulance would take 20 minutes to get to his house at least."

"True. When you put it that way. So he'll actually be in here on nasal O2 here by the time the EMTs fininish their coffee."

"There's a girl with experience."

"A woman with experience, Dr. Galen."

"Looks like a girl to me."

"Thanks."

While I'm standing at the telephone, I dial 237-5492 again.

"Pharmacist."

"Hi, Dr. Moore. Galen again. Anything happen?"

"Yeah. I told her I would fill the prescription, but it would take a little while, I had to send out. She waited for, oh, fifteen minutes. Front-office clerk says she saw a card in the girl's wallet. Says the name wasn't Wanda Edwards. The police did come, but she was gone before they showed up."

"Too bad."

"Yeah. I gave them a description, but even if they caught her the case would be hard for the DA to do anything with. Probably end up a misdemeanor or a dropped charge. They may call you. Probably not."

"Well, thanks for your efforts. The bad news is she'll probably try it again."

"Yeah, but there's some good news. . . she won't try it with you or me."

I hang up the phone. "Whatever else happens I'm going to ICU Green and see about Randolph -- now," I announce to anyone who's listening.

Nobody apparently is.

HARDWARE/SOFTWARE

I take the shortcut through X-ray. There are several patients on stretchers lined up in the hall, one in a wheelchair. Some are waiting for X-rays. Some are waiting to confirm that their films, just taken, are technically adequate. None are smiling.

I cut through the OR suite, another shortcut. You're not supposed to do that -- sterility and all. I open the wide door to ICU Green and see that things are buzzing. And I see that all is not well, because Gloria is standing outside Randolph's room, mouth pouting, both hands on both hips.

"You're not going to believe this, Dr. Galen."

"Just give it to me all at once."

"You know, they had to modify the plumbing in all the ICU rooms to handle the outflow from the kidney."

"Sure. Took an act of Congress."

"Well, there's one room out of 18 that didn't make it."

"Let me guess -- the one Randolph's in."

"You got it. The maintenance man is on the way."

"That won't cut it. It'll take him hours to change those fittings. Let's move Randolph."

"There aren't any empty ICU rooms."

"Then we'll swap."

Pauline, the head nurse of ICU Green, has jet black hair, translucent green eyes, luminous ivory skin, and a worried expression. "That's against policy in the ICU suites, Dr. Galen. We'd have to call the resource nurse and she'd have to call the administrator."

"Tell you what. Have someone call the resource nurse. Tell her Dr. Galen is in here changing beds around like crazy. Tell her to call the administrator, Congress, the police, the doctor, you can't do a thing with Dr. Galen. Where's a bed where the patient isn't on the ventilator?"

"Number three. She's just on a monitor."

"Let's swap. Now."

I personally explain to the poor confused elderly lady in ICU Green Room 3 that we have an emergency requiring

303

specialized equipment which is only available in her cubicle.
I carefully do not tell her that it's a goddam drain pipe.

Changing beds sounds easier than it is. You have the
oxygen line, the monitor line, the IV lines, the poles, the cord
for the electric bed. There's never enough room or enough
people. Then we encounter another problem.

"The power cord for the kidney won't plug in here,"
Gloria tells me.

"Whady'a mean, there's no place to plug it in?"

"Right. And you can't use a multiple plug system, it'll
overload the circuit with all this equipment."

"Damn," I respond.

"Shit," suggests Pauline. Then she raises her
shoulders and covers her mouth.

"Unplug the power bed," I tell Gloria.

"Then he'll have to lie flat all the time."

"There's a manual mechanism to raise the bed."

"I didn't know that. How do you work it?" asks
Pauline.

"Damn if I know. This is the time to call the maintenance people. Get them over here. Tell them to bring the
directions. We may even break down and read the damn
instructions. What 's Randolph's pressure?"

"Eighty systolic."

"What about the tracing?"

"Looking a little worse. QRS wider."

"Put Randolph down flat. Then get four extra pillows
under him. If the hardware's not working, use the software.

"And turn the goddamn kidney on."

THE STING

CALL # 17 - 11:18 - 233-9886 - JANE BOSTWICK -
BEE STING REACTION

This could be serious -- acute anaphylaxis, if it occurs, can be fatal within minutes. I use one of the the ICU desk phones. The line is busy. I call the operator. The phone rings and rings. Unusual to get a bee sting this time of night.

"Can I help you?"

"Yes, This is Doctor Galen. I have an emergency. Could you interrupt the call on this line, please: 233-9886."

"I'll see if there is a conversation on the line."

Pause.

"There *is* a conversation on that line."

"Yes, great. Can you interrupt it, please?"

"You're saying this is an emergency."

"It sure is."

"And you're a doctor."

"Yes."

"I am required to ask you if you are aware of the penalty for falsely declaring an emergency in order to interrupt a private telephone call."

"I am aware it's against the law. I don't know the penalty. Are you aware of what I'm going to do if this patient dies because of all this bullshit?"

"I'll connect you, sir, but foul language is not necessary. As a matter of fact, it's against the law to use foul language on the telephone."

305

"Nothing else has worked."

"What?"

"Can you just please connect me?"

"I'll break in on the line and have the party hang up. Then I'll dial and patch you in."

"Thanks."

Pause. Then the phone at the other end rings.

"Hello," says a woman's voice, in no apparent distress.

"Here's your party," says the operator. "Doctor, would you give me your name and telephone number again please?"

"So you can report me to my Boy Scout leader? I give the information. Mrs. Bostwick?"

"Yes. Dr. Galen?"

"I understand you've had a bee sting reaction. What's happening to you?"

"Well, I was stung two days ago."

"Two *days* ago?"

"Yes. Out in the yard. It hurt at first, then it got better."

"Yes?"

"And during the afternoon it's kind of swollen up and gotten red."

"Does it hurt, or itch?"

"Mostly itches."

"You just have the typical delayed reaction to a beesting, Mrs. Bostwick. Shows up at about 48 hours. I'd put some ice on it and take an antihistamine every four hours for

306

the next day or so. Do you have any Benadryl or Chlortrimeton?"

"Benadryl. You know, that you get over-the-counter."

"Yes. 25 milligrams. Take one every four hours while you're awake."

"Is this a dangerous reaction, Doctor?"

"No, ma'am. The only dangerous kind is the immediate reaction -- within the first five minutes. This is a nuisance reaction, should be better tomorrow, gone the next day."

"Good. Thanks very much for calling."

"You're welcome. Oh, and Mrs. Bostwick -- " *Why didn't you call earlier today? And don't you know that when we get a beep this time of night we assume it's urgent, we break our necks to get through? And why did you put in a call and then get on the damn telephone?*

"Yes, Doctor?"

"Uh -- let us know if things don't improve." *Us,* objective case of *We.*

"I will. Thanks again."

PAIN IN A SPECIAL PLACE

Janet hands me another clipboard. "Woman named Egbert. Abdominal pain. She's in 8."

"Janet, are you my private duty nurse now? I hope."

"No, Dr. Galen, but you do seem to be the main show here tonight."

"What happened to the lady in the accident with the pelvic pain and hypotension and so forth – Billie?"

"Fine. Well, she's got pelvic fractures. Blood pressure's OK now. A lot of pain. The orthopods admitted her. Findlay, I think. Dr. Vinson sewed up her lacerations. Her boyfriend's not so good. Cervical fracture but no apparent cord injury. He's in tongs."

Tongs. Crutchfield tongs -- surely the most medieval of all modern contrivances. In order to immobilize the neck of someone with a spinal fracture they bore holes in the outer tables of the skull and stick tongs in the holes and then put traction on the device. Like the old-fashioned things they used for block ice. They do that until a definitive fusion procedure can be done on the spine. The patient looks like the victim of a barbarian insurrection who resisted the pain of the rack; so he is now moved to the next stage of torture in order to induce a confession. But the paradox is complete: the tongs cause no pain and they rescue him from the worst torture of all -- lifelong paralysis from the neck down.

"Yeah, abdominal pain. Mrs. Egbert. She called earlier. We'll need a CBC and urine at least. I'll look in and get started, but we've got a possible infarct coming."

"You mentioned the lab earlier -- it's already drawn. Also they're holding blood for a 6 and whatever."

"Good."

June Egbert seems placid enough lying on the stretcher in Room 8. She has sort of ash-blond hair, the kind you know is always natural because nobody dyes it that color. She has fine, catlike features which, cosmetically speaking,

308

work out very well. I introduce myself to her and her husband. He says his name is Raymond. He never takes his eyes from his wife.

"How did this come on, Mrs. Egbert?"

"My whole stomach was kind of queasy this morning and then it started hurting here --" She indicates the mid upper abdominal area, which doctors call the epigastrium.

"Have you thrown up?"

"After lunch. Once. Then I didn't want any supper."

"And now. Where does it hurt the most now? Same place?"

"No. Now it hurts right here." She places her hand on the right lower portion of the abdomen, identified in medical geography as the right lower quadrant.

"If you had to take two fingers --" I pick up her index and forefinger in my hand -- "and put them on the most painful spot, where would you point?"

"Here, I guess." She touches a spot midway between the navel and the hipbone. On the medical record I will later refer to this spot as "equidistant from the umbilicus and the anterior superior iliac spine."

And even the newest freshman medical student would recognize this spot as McBurney's Point. Now McBurney's Point is not a picnic area on the ocean. It is the place which generally speaking overlies the appendix, and, so far, June Egbert is making her bid for a classic textbook case of acute appendicitis.

And that in itself is a problem.

As gently as possible I explore various parts of her abdomen with my right hand, the left positioned on top. The examining physician (if right-handed) is supposed to let the right hand remain relaxed, sensitive, perceptive while he applies pressure with the left. I start with the distant Left Upper Quadrant, which proves slack and non-tender. Then the Left Lower Quadrant. Then the RUQ.

And now, very gingerly, I touch the area which immortalizes Dr. McBurney. Even the vaguest pressure causes her to wince, bring up her right leg, lift her head from the stretcher, and tighten the abdominal muscles in that area -- so tightly, in fact, that her RLQ feels like a tabletop. I increase the pressure slightly. She winces more. Then, abruptly, I take my hand away.

"Ow!" June cries out and sits up.

"Sorry, Mrs. Egbert, I have to do this. That last little manuever was to show what we call rebound tenderness."

"It's OK, Doctor. What have I got, appendicitis?"

"Sure acting that way. When was your last period?"

"Started, let's see, about, when, two weeks ago?" She looks at Raymond. Raymond is still looking at her.

"About then," Raymond says.

"Lasted about five days, didn't it?" she asks.

"Stopped on a Monday." Raymond's eyes have never left her.

I look at Mr. Egbert and then back at June. "No reason to suspect you're pregnant?"

"No, no. I don't think so. We haven't been using any contraceptives, but . . . ."

310

"No birth control pills?"

"No. Not since, oh, six months ago."

"Stopped on April 14," says Raymond.

Improbable as it seems, I know that pregnancy can occur with no interruption of periods. And it can occur sometimes not in its rightful place in the uterus but in the Fallopian tube. If it occurs in the tube on the right, it can look for all the world like appendicitis. And I know too about *mittelschmerz* -- rupture of an ovarian cyst. This characteristically occurs at the time of ovulation, about midway in the cycle.

"OK. We'll see what the white count is, check the urine, even do a pregnancy test just for good measure. You still need a pelvic and rectal examination. Right now we need a surgeon to see you. Do you have one, or know one you'd like to see?"

The Egberts eyes meet. "Well, we know Dr. Randall at church," says Mr. Egbert. "Is he good?"

"Excellent. But I think his partner, Dr. Barton, is on call tonight. He's top-drawer, too. Shall I call him?"

"Yes, please, Doctor, if he's your choice," says June.

Janet comes in and puts her hand on my arm. "The chest pain is here. In 12. Looks pretty -- sick. We're doing the usual."

"OK. Janet, get somebody to call Dr. Barton. Tell him possible appendix. Go ahead with the six and get a pregnancy test too. Be sure to tell Barton Mrs. Egbert hasn't had a pelvic or rectal yet, and I haven't had time to write anything down yet . . . anywhere."

311

PAIN IN THE CHEST

Henry Adams is easy. That is, his diagnosis. Lying on the stretcher in Room 12 with his head elevated to 30 degrees, he is pale, sweaty, scared-looking, and holds his right hand over his breastbone. He already has an IV going, oxygen in his nose, the monitor on his chest, and the automatic BP cuff on his arm. His electrocardiogram looks like this:

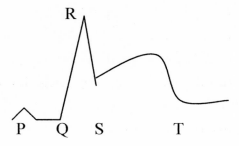

The critical findings are his ST segments, which are markedly elevated in leads 2, 3, AVF, and depressed in 1 and AVR. Normally they would be "isoelectric"; that is, on the same level with the rest of the baseline.

So, Henry Adams is easy -- the diagnosis, that is: acute inferior myocardial infarction in progress. As a matter of fact, "STEMI – ST Elevation Myocardial Infarction" – which is much discussed in the medical literature and has a special method of recommended treatment.

And Henry Adams' treatment will be complicated indeed.

"A lot of pain, Mr. Adams?"

"Yeah, a lot. Started getting worse in the car."

The monitor shows pulse 94, BP 110/76. "Let's give him morphine 3 milligrams IV now, then repeat in ten minutes if no big change. Henry," (it's time to drop the formality) "have you ever had a bleeding ulcer, or any bleeding from your intestinal tract?"

"No, sir."

"Tendency to bleed abnormally anywhere?"

"No."

"Never had a stroke?"

"Not yet."

"You're, let's see, 42?"

"Yes, in June."

"No real medical problems? Diabetes? High blood pressure?"

"No, nothing. Until this."

"Janet -- where's Janet?"

"I'm working this room, Dr. Galen."

"Oh, yes, David, sure, how are you. David -- let's activate the protocol."

"TPA?"

"Right. TPA. Stat."

Janet's head appears at the door. "Somebody to see you outside, Dr. Galen."

"To see me?"

"Yes. A doctor."

"What doctor?"

"Your son."

"Tell him to come in. OK, David, we'll have to get all the clotting studies, get four IVs going and so forth. Henry, we'll need a cardiologist to help us. Want me to pick one?"

"Yessir, please, whoever you think."

"David -- no, keep on with what you're doing. Janet, you still there?"

Janine speaks up. "No, but *I* am, Dr. Galen."

"Good, Janine. Get Dr. Wasatch or Wanamaker on the line, whoever's on call for the cardiology group. Tell him we've got an acute inferior, we're starting TPA. We'd all love to see him."

"How's it going, Dad?" John Galen, Jr., MD, joins us at the bedside. He has on tan corduroy pants and a light green canvas shirt with the sleeves rolled up.

"Not too bad, Johnny, er, John. Henry, this is my son, Dr. Galen. Some of us call him Dr. Boy."

Dr. Boy does not appear to consider the last statement hilarious.

"Glad to meet you," says Henry Adams, weakly offering his hand.

"Same here, sir. Bet you'll be feeling better soon." Dr. Boy shakes Henry's hand and turns to me. "Hear things have been moving right along over here. Happened to call in about Mrs. Dunbar's blood sugar up on 5 West and they said you were admitting them right and left."

"Enough to keep us occupied. So what're you doing here, you're not on call. What happened, tired of working in your gun workshop?"

"Naw, the router broke down."

314

"At what, midnight?" I look at my watch. It says 11:56.

"Whatever. Got any more chores?"

"Let's step outside."

"I do have a few items to follow up on, Johnny. And then there's about six more calls in this thing. Tell you what, since you've offered." I hold up the grey cigarette package. "You get your choice of this or Henry Adams."

"That's easy."

"It is?"

"Yep. Henry, here I come."

For a young physician just out of training, a battlefield case like Henry Adams is nirvana; a list of phone calls of dubious urgency is anathema. Indeed, with Henry Adams' heart attack, Dr. Boy has now been consigned to home ground. He will perform with aplomb. He will swim around amid monitors and IV tubing and rhythm strips and electrolytes in languid comfort. He will not take the short cuts which older practitioners like myself have learned are available -- the cursory neurological exam, the rapid survey of the review of systems, the omission of repetitive blood gases. He will do everything in excruciating and ritualistic detail.

I would have missed nothing important.

He will miss nothing at all.

Most of the young physicians are cut from the same bolt. But new emergency room doctors are something special: they will decorate the simplest case with an elaborate

315

biochemical and radiographic filigree before calling the attending physician.

As if to prove the point, Tom Vinson walks up with an apologetic expression and a full clipboard. "Got a woman here with chest pain, Dr. Galen. We've worked her up but nothing is very definite. Mind taking a look at her?"

"Just what I need, Tom. Sure, I'll see her. But I may get interrupted by one of my other victims."

"It's OK, I know you're crunched here. She doesn't look that sick. But she's been here about three hours."

Ginger intercepts me. "Dr. Galen -- telephone -- the AT &T operator."

"I can' t talk now."

"Then she says can I give you a message?"

"Give it."

"Says she's sorry she had to delay you with company procedure earlier."

"Yeah, right. Did she call my scout leader?"

"What? What scout leader? Wants to know if the patient is okay. She's worried. Is the woman going to be all right?"

"Tell her the patient will be okay. And tell her --"

"Yes, Dr. Galen?"

"Tell her I'm sorry I said *bullshit*."

Ginger laughs ruefully, but Ginger, I know, is not insulted; such verbiage is the common coin of her generation. "Dr. Galen, you don't want me to tell her that."

316

"Well, let's see then. Just tell her thanks for calling back. And, Ginger --"

"Yessir."

"Tell her -- tell her thanks for worrying."

PAIN IN THE CHEST, ANOTHER VERSION

I finally get to Jane Sing, an attractive young Asian woman wearing a tailored grey suit, a white blouse, and a solid dark blue cravat, who tells me she has had a catching type pain in her left lower chest for most of the day. She says it comes and goes, gets intense, then disappears again.

I look at her workup: complete blood count, urinalysis, biochemical profile, including 21 separate determinations, amylase, chest x-ray, electrocardiogram, even a nuclear lung scan. Everything is perfectly normal. This is all reassuring, of course: the tests tend to rule out such things as heart attack, pneumothorax, pulmonary embolism, pancreatitis, pneumonia, pleurisy with effusion, lung tumor, fractured ribs, ruptured esophagus, hepatitis, and perforated peptic ulcer. Great.

But let's be reasonable. This 34-year old Chinese woman is at a vanishingly low risk for heart attack -- she's young, she's female, she's Asian, she's lean, has normal blood pressure, no diabetes, and the pain is of the wrong type, in the wrong place. There is no reason to think of clots breaking off and going to her lungs. Nothing on examination remotely suggests anything wrong in the abdomen. She hasn't the picture for a perforated esophagus. The pain is episodic and "pleuritic" in nature. The season is fall.

317

As I say, let's be reasonable: she has pleurodynia.

This is a painful but harmless infection with one of the enteroviruses known as Coxsackie. The bug, I know, is going around anyway, just as it did among the children in the school epidemic in Coxsackie, New York, a town which gave the virus its name. Like the schoolchildren, Jane has the gripping pain from inflammation of diaphragmatic muscle characteristic of the disease. She needs relief of pain and reassurance, not three hours of investigation and a $1500 bill.

I ruminate that, left to my own devices in the office, I would have examined her, probably gotten a chest x-ray, and given her Tylenol with codeine and an anti-inflammatory drug. That would have been it: maybe $80. But then 30 years of seeing patients, many before sophisticated procedures became readily available, have created intuitive patterns in the mental matrix of docs my age that make pleurodynia and a thousand other clinical syndromes as reflexly recognizable as an old friend in the marketplace.

Tom Vinson hasn't gotten there yet. And Tom faces another specter with which he has not yet made his peace: malpractice. What if, he says to himself. What if she has a lung tumor and I miss it? A pulmonary embolus? Could I defend myself in court without having done a lung scan? Some estimate that 35% of the massive $1.9 trillion national health bill is attributable to this defensive dread of being consigned to the public stocks.

I too know that every single patient contact is a potential suit. Particularly in the emergency setting. Particularly with a patient whom I don't know, whom I'm seeing for the first time. Of course, we are all insured, but more importantly I have now become *inured*. I cannot live and work with a phantom judge or a jury -- both untrained in medicine -- peering over my shoulder. My credo has finally evolved: I will do my best. I will do what is indicated. I will not decorate the chart with delicate and expensive gilding. I will treat my patient and my conscience. I will not treat the courts.

"We call this pleurodynia, Ms. Sing. Sort of like pleurisy. It's a virus. It will hurt a few days and then go away. It's not serious. I'll give you some medication to relieve the pain and inflammation. Antibiotics don't help this."

"That's all it is?"

"Yes. Not pneumonia or a collapsed lung or a heart attack or anything like that."

"That's a relief. I didn't know what was happening, it hurt so much."

And then, I want to give her something for her time and trouble and expense. So I say, "And all these procedures -- you can take some consolation from them."

"How do you mean, Doctor?"

"You don't have much of anything wrong with you -- you've passed all these tests with flying colors."

"That's good. I'm sure glad I had everything done."

319

Glad you had everything done? I start back to tell Tom about the disposition of this patient. But I guess I won't tell him about the credo.

He may not be ready yet.

APPENDICITIS . . .MAYBE

"Dr. Galen, you got an overhead page from 5 North." Ginger stands in the bay, this time with her head tilted wistfully, her left hand in one of her many pants pockets. "I answered it, it's Celeste. Said she's been beeping you for 30 minutes, they've had a death up there, one of Dr. Fitz's patients."

"Thought you were monitoring my beeper."

"You took it back."

"Oh." I look down. Indeed, it is at my belt. "Well, did they code her?"

"No. She was a No Ward."

"Family up there?"

"Didn't say."

"OK, I'll go now. Got to check on Minnie and Randolph anyway. Dr. Barton ever come?"

"He just came out of Mrs. Egbert's room and called the operating room."

"That tells you something. What was her white count?"

"Let's see . . .here it is. . . 16,500 -- high."

Earl Barton walks up. "Pretty classic appendix," he says.

"Kind of worries me," I offer. "Too perfect."

"No problem. Yeah." He chuckles. "Probably turn out to be something weird. Or maybe nothing. Anyway, with those findings we sure got to look."

"Right. Sorry we had to call you at this hour, and sorry I had someone else call you, I was fighting alligators. "

"Way it goes. Do 'em when we see 'em. Appreciate the call."

But 1 a. m., I know, is the worst possible hour for a case of this kind. At eight p. m. the surgeon can come in, evaluate the patient, prepare him or her for surgery, go to the OR, finish up, and be in bed by midnight -- and get six hours of sleep before another full day. Or five a. m. -- he just gets an early start. But 1 a. m. -- too early to defer surgery for the morning hours, just right to rob him of a night's rest. Rest he'll never catch up on. But as Earl Barton says, way it goes.

And acute appendicitis: the simplest, clearest surgical diagnosis and the most straightforward surgical cure, right? Maybe. Or -- the most complex, the most convoluted, and the most tragically complicated. It has been classically preached that one out of five appendectomies should produce a normal appendix: a pronouncement designed to insure that no true appendicitis is missed. Better to do an occasional unnecessary operation, it is said, than risk perforation of a hot appendix, with attendant peritonitis, sepsis, abcess formation. Newer and more careful diagnostic techniques have reduced this negative rate to about 6-8%. But a long list of other things can simulate the picture: acute gastroenteritis, particularly with bugs called *Yersinia* and *Helicobacter*;

321

ruptured ovarian cyst; "mesenteric adenitis" (viral inflammation of the lymph nodes in the abdominal cavity); regional enteritis (Crohn's disease), tubal pregnancy, and so on. But soon Earl will find out for sure and June Egbert will be on safe ground. With a two-inch wound in her right lower quadrant.

Some are minimizing the wound these days -- they do a laparoscopic procedure in which a one-half inch incision just below the navel is substituted for the traditional approach, and a long fiberoptic seeing-eye tube probes around and does the job. Many surgeons do not think this is the right way to proceed: what if it's something else? what if there's a leak, a little abscess? And the old adage persists in some quarters: "Small incision, small surgeon." Time will tell about technique. Meanwhile June Egbert will be getting the old- fashioned treatment.

INTENSIVE/EXPENSIVE

I go to intensive care first, the pronouncing will have to wait. Follow the rule: the quick before the dead.

Intensive care is sometimes called extensive care, expensive care. Both are accurate. One of my patients recently slipped and said "insensitive care." But that's not true -- you get the best attention in the world there.

I reflect on the fact that these units are labeled Red, Blue, and Green rather than something like A, B, and C; this is, of course, diagnostic of the fact that women named them. And the selection of costumes clearly identify the largely

female nursing service, rather than the largely male medical
staff, as the authors of dress code. They wear emerald in
Green, cobalt in Blue, and a sort of cerise-maroon in Red.
Doctors would have probably decreed all white in all three
and maybe called the units Mach I, Mach II, Mach III. Vive
la difference.

Randolph Brown is giggling, if a 300-pound man can
giggle, and Gloria, the dialysis nurse, is smiling broadly as I
walk into Room 3 of ICU Green.

"What's happening, you folks thinking of joining the
plumbers' union?"

"You got it Doctor. Now that's funny too." He
giggles some more.

"Fill me in," I suggest.

"He means -- well, the drain is working," Gloria says.
"But we were talking about another kind of plumbing, weren't
we, Randolph?"

"Yeah," he says. "I was asking Gloria here, when I
get a kidney transplant, what if I get a woman's kidney. And
she says, it will work as well as a man's. But, I said, will I
have to sit down to pee the rest of my life? And she says
probably. And I said it will be hell in the woods deer-
hunting. And she said don't worry, the other boys will think
it's cute."

"The big problem," I say, "will be getting to the deer
preserve in the first place. You'll have to stop at every service
station."

"Now *that*, " Gloria says, "isn't funny."

"Yeah," says Randolph. "You ain't a male whatchamacallit pig, are you, Doctor Galen?"

"Once in a while I'm accused of that."

"You know how to tell, don't you?"

"How?"

"If there's only one john and you leave the toilet seat up."

Gloria now turns her head aside and shakes it hopelessly. The gesture says That's enough now, boys. Indeed, an outsider might wonder why all this patter in the first place. Isn't this a serious moment, an emergency, not a time to be horsing around? Aren't we worried about this man dying, shouldn't we be finding out if his potassium is down?

But, you see, we have. The machine is running smoothly, the drain is fixed, the potassium, we know, is one of the first things to come pouring out with the artificial kidney. Once you're up and running, things have to get better. Most important, Randolph and Gloria are joking. So his circulatory dynamics are restored, his brain is getting plenty of blood, his *angor animi* has dissipated. It is a crucial clinical fact for me to know that he is comfortable enough to tell jokes.

And the monitors tell the same story. The automatic BP cuff device, now set to inflate every five minutes, says 142/76, up from previously. The cardiac monitor says pulse 104: his potassium-poisoned slow rate has now speeded up. I look at the LED display of cardiac rhythm but, being old-fashioned, press the button for a printout of the precordial lead. It looks much better.

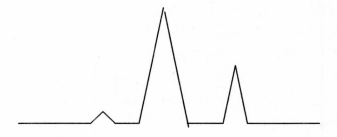

And only 30 minutes after starting dialysis.

"How's your breathing, Randolph?"

"A lot better, Doc."

"Do you still feel weak?"

"A little washed-out. But okay."

"How's your muscle strength?"

"Pretty good, I think." He pulls himself up as if to demonstrate.

"Watch it, Randolph. All these lines," cautions Gloria.

As I examine his chest, I note the two lengths of plastic tubing leading to a site just below Randolph's left collarbone. One is marked with a red sleeve, the other with a blue one. The red is for "arterial": that is, blood coming out of Randolph; the blue is for "venous": blood returning to him. They both lead to a Y-connector which converges into a single line the size of the straw you use for a Big Mac Frosty. This straw enters the skin and passes into the left subclavian vein and then into the superior vena cava. It may even extend all the way into the right side of the heart.

325

"Where's his post-procedure film, Gloria?"

"Outside on the viewbox,. The line's in good position, the tip is in the right atrium. We're getting good flow. No sign of pneumothorax."

Gloria has just reassured me that the chief complication of inserting a subclavian catheter – collapsed lung-- did not occur.

The other end of the arterial and venous lines lead to the artificial kidney complex. The red line leads to a rotary pump, which squeezes the blood along to enter the dialytic cartridge, referred to as "the kidney." Here blood passes into the ends of hundreds of tiny hollow fibers, like hairs. The dialysis bath, fluid of ideal composition, flows in the opposite direction around the hairs, to wit:

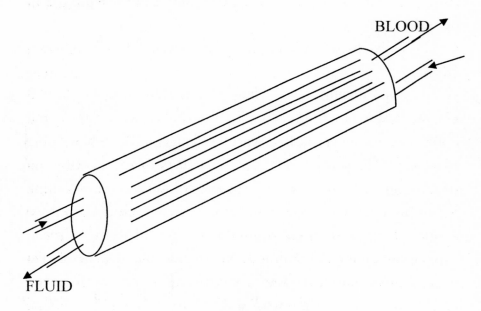

BLOOD

FLUID

The plasma of the blood tends to equilibrate with the ideal bath fluid as it passes along the hair. At the entry point the blood, with its distorted composition, enters the fiber. It contains poisons, like urea, and indols, and phenols, and imidazoles. And in Randolph's case, too much $K+$. Along the way, water, and urea, and potassium, and what-have-you pass back and forth through the membrane, becoming equalized on either side. Only the blood proteins have big enough molecules to remain inside the hair, and the force they exert, called osmotic pressure, is what keeps all the water of plasma from oozing out. At the exit point, then, the blood is in better shape than it was to start with, having been in better company along the course of the hair. This blood eventually returns to Randolph. Each minute of dialysis processes 200 to 400 milliliters (a glassful to a pint) of blood; each minute Randolph gets a little better.

I look at the gauges and dials and switches and alarms all over the face of the kidney machine --the Hanover Hemodial, the very latest thing. You can ratchet in the amount of fluid you want to remove by altering the transmembrane pressure. You can request a given flow rate. You can stop dialysis entirely, keep the blood flowing on bypass. If you need only to remove fluid, you can stop the bath flow and "suck" fluid out of the blood. Want to lose 10 pounds (of fluid, that is) in three hours? Dial it in. You can change the venous pressure, dictate the $K+$ concentration, set the alarms for any parameter. In three hours, it's over.

We have come a long way, baby. In the old days, the fifties, when the artificial kidney was first being tried, it took

327

three doctors and three nurses -- all capable of heavy lifting -- eight hours to carry off the whole procedure. The machine, known as the Kolff-Brigham kidney, was the size of two oil drums end-to-end, slowly rotating in a vat the size of two bathtubs. You had to make up the bath as you went -- add 50 grams of sodium, 12 grams of calcium, etc. The blood sleeve was enormous and wrapped around and around the whole drum; it required four units of blood to fill it. Fluid balance was uncontrollable. The patient might gain or lose weight, would likely have seizures. You didn't use this contraption very often -- only in patients who seemed to be in temporary kidney failure and only when they looked pretty desperate.

Not that everything nowadays is automatic. The patient may drop his blood pressure out when he goes on the machine. The subclavian lines may not work. The venous pressure may skyrocket. The blood may clot -- you lose a pint of blood in the machine and have to replace everything. The patient may bleed somewhere as a result of the heparin you have to use as an anticoagulant. He may be or become delirious and, in spite of restraints, jerk out the lines.

But things usually go well and that's the case with Randolph. His blood pressure has come up to baseline. His pulse, depressed by the potassium intoxication, is back to normal. His lungs, congested and causing respiratory distress, are clearing perceptibly. His oxygen saturation is above 92%. The QRS complex of his EKG has narrowed, the P waves have returned, the T wave is coming down. The potassium level in the blood --

"K+ is 6.0 now, Dr. Galen."

The immediate threat of cardiac arrest is over, and circulatory dynamics are greatly improved. All these indices are fine, but, you see, the single index which reflects the normalization of all these variables in Randolph's case was already in plain view to the observant nurse and clinician.

That is, a 300-pound man, at 9 p. m. in fear of his life, at 1 a. m. was giggling.

WAXING, WANING

Minnie Jones is sitting up on the side of her bed in Room 324, feet propped on the lowered siderails, eating an apple. She is looking at her reflection in the mirror, turning her head this way and that, smiling and grimacing, just checking. To me her smiles and grimaces look pretty normal. The heparin drip is going, each drop of the powerful anticoagulant monitored by the IMED, an obsessive-compulsive device conceived to ration jealously every critical dollop. It is an elongated gray box with lights and dials mounted on an IV stand. It looks like a sentinel with a life of its own.

Minnie sees me and smiles broadly. Both sides of her face move very well. She shakes her head. "Cain't get nothin' to eat roun' here, Doctor. Sister brought me this here apple. Better'n nothin.'"

"You weren't supposed to be eating yet, Minnie, until we saw how this stroke was going to behave. We'll get you some food soon. Want a snack?"

"Anythin', Doctor."

"How do you feel?"

329

"Feels fine."

"No weakness now?"

"Nossir. Not right now. Had a little flittin' spell on the way up to the room."

"Let the nurses know if you have any more flittin' spells or need anything. You know how to use the buzzer?

"They say all you has to do is press this here bar on the little clicker thing."

"That's right. Let them know if you want them. They'll be checking on you anyway, maybe more than you want them to. Your sister go home?

"Yessir. She had to practice with the church choir."

"Fine. See you later."

I walk to the 3-Center nursing station and pick up Minnie's chart. I look at the orders I wrote in the emergency room:

ORDERS

Diagnosis: Transient Ischemic Attacks
Condition: Serious
1. NPO x clear liquids until further notice
2. BR c BRP with assistance
3. VS & Neuro Checks q 4h
4. I & O q 8 h.
5. Daily weights & rec
5 a. Accuchecks q 4 h and record.
5 b. Sliding scale: # units reg Humulin-R q 4 h = BS -100/30. No insulin if under 200
<u>*Already done in ER:*</u>
6. CBC, SMA-6, PT, PTT ua, stat
7. SMA - 12 "now"
8. Chest PA & lat stat; head CT s contrast
9. 12-lead EKG stat
10. Aq heparin 4000 units stat IV bolus -- given at 1118 hours

11. D - 5 - W 1000 ml c 10,000 u aq heparin to run at 100 ml/h to deliver1000
u heparin /h - started at 1134 hrs
<u>Other orders:</u>
12. Follow standard heparin protocol
13. Colace 100 mg daily
14. MOM 45 ml HS prn constipation
15. Benadryl 50 mg hs prn sleep
16. Non-invasive carotid duplex studies in a. m.
17. Echocardiogram in a. m.
18. Will get neuro consult in a. m.
   --John Galen, MD

Now, the powers-that-be are getting ready to put this all on the computer as the hospital moves to a "paperless" system. The Institute of Medicine wants this, industry wants it, and now the government is beginning to insist on it. But you won't be able to take the chart into the rooms, then. Will a line form to get to the computers? The main thing most paperless systems I've seen generate is -- huge amounts of paper. We shall see, we shall see.

   What my orders really mean:
   1. Nothing by mouth except clear liquids (stroke patients may have problems swallowing, and food down the windpipe is much to be avoided)
   2. Bed rest with bathroom privileges . . .
   3. Vital signs (temperature, pulse, respiration, blood pressure) and neurological evaluation every four hours. The neuro checks include mental status ("Do you know where you are and why, Minnie?"), pupil size and reaction, ability to move extremities normally, etc.
   4. Intake and output of liquids every eight hours
   5. Weigh the patient daily and record
5 a and b were obviously squeezed in later:
   5 a. Fingerstick blood sugar determinations every four hours
   5 b. Every time a blood sugar value is obtained by the accucheck technique, take the number and subtract 100 (normal blood sugar) from it, then divide that by 30 and give that number of units of reglar human insulin

subcutaneously. (So, if the accucheck says 370, you subtract 100. That's 270; divided by 30, that's 9 units)

6.   Complete blood count, part of the biochemical profile, prothrombin time, partial thromboplastin time (both measures of blood clotting), urinalysis -- right away

7.   Remainder of biochemical profile -- as soon as possible

8.   Chest X-ray, including postero-anterior and lateral views -- right away; computerized tomography of head and brain, not using contrast material ("dye")

9.   Electrocardiogram with all 12 directions -- right away

10.   Aqueous heparin 1000 units given right away as a single injection into the vein . . .

11.   Five-percent dextrose in sterile distilled water, 1000 milliliters with 10,000 units of aqueous heparin, to run at 100 millliliters an hour so as to infuse 1000 units of the heparin each hour . . .

12.   The standard heparin protocol is a page of single-spaced typewritten instructions on how to govern the heparin infusion, based on checking the degree of blood-thinning using periodic PTT checks, then regulating the IMED administration device.   This plan, like all cookbook schemes, assumes every patient is the same.   Since in fact every patient is different, the doctor must stand by and tailor the program, as in this case, to Minnie.

13.   A stool softener

14.   None other than milk of magnesia, an ounce and a half at the hour of sleep as needed for constipation

15.   A common antihistamine, here used for sedation -- stronger agents are usually avoided in patients with neurological problems to avoid confusing the mental picture

16.   Tests which "listen" for turbulence over the carotid arteries in the neck, envision the interior of the arteries with sonar waves, and indirectly measure the pressure in them by estimating the amount of force it requires to stop the pulsations in the retinal vessels.

17.   A sonar image of the heart as it contracts and relaxes.   It paints a picture of the valves, tells if they leak, and visualizes the chambers, looking for any clots within.

18.   A neurologist will be summoned to provide consultation.

Now I write:

Soft diet, 1800 cal ADA -- please obtain HS snack tonight

332

(This means 1800-calorie diet as outlined by the American Diabetic Association -- please obtain a bedtime snack)

Minnie is holding her own; maybe brain damage can be averted. Tomorrow we'll do some studies searching for the source of her little platelet plug -- the carotid arteries? the heart? or the small vessels of the brain itself? We'll have the neurologists see her, but I'm sure we've carried out the essentials they'd recommend at this stage. I guess I'm doing all I can now.

Although, come to think of it, the hospital chapel is right on my way.

PRONOUNCING

"The family is in there, Dr. Galen," says Celeste. "They seem to be handling it pretty well."

You can read the empathy on Celeste's face. Her perfect white skin is suffused with a pink glow below the deep mahogany of her slightly rumpled wedge-cut hair. There is a mistiness in her outsize caramel eyes. She is not sorry that Mrs. Atterman is gone, for the situation was hopeless and the patient was miserable, but Celeste feels every pulse of grief, of guilt, of the family. She has, I know, been standing in the room with them, helping to absorb the unexpected shock of reality. For every death, no matter how expected, even desired, is surprising in the very way it brings surprise.

333

Celeste is, I think, pretty typical of most RNs. You may hear that the nursing profession isn't what it used to be. They aren't as caring, don't spend enough time with the patient, are trying to take over the doctors' function, hang out at the desk instead of the bedside. It's true that the administrative burden has accelerated mightily -- more forms to fill out, reports to file. You must, you see, document everything. Completing the Care Plan alone -- an extensive computerized packet on every patient -- is an absorbing task. Yet almost no one, save perhaps the inspecting agencies, even looks at them. Certainly not the doctors; they go straight to the hand-written notes or, better, ask the nurses how the patient is doing. Of course, the same pattern is pervading all aspects of the health-care system. I sometimes think here at Metro we will soon have two hospitals with two staffs -- one to do the work, one to watch the others and write up the reports. Document, document. If you're one of the working half, you step around the observers, the documentarians, and get things done the best you can while the ball-points scratch and the laser printers grind.

No, the nurses aren't what they used to be: they're better. A lot better. They are smarter, better trained, more committed, more caring. They have more to do and do it superbly. At times, like now, I think Celeste and her breed of career nurses are the possibly the finest people on earth, a chosen clan -- dedicated to the unobtrusive performance of their tasks, ignoring the rigors of their schedule, the whips of unthinking doctors and the scorns of demanding family members.

I remember, not long ago, on 3 South, a tiny brunette nurse named Linda, about 24 years old; she saw me and turned away, mopping her eyes with a Kleenex.

"I'm sorry, Dr. Galen. I shouldn't be this way. It's just Mrs. Bainbridge -- she's so sick with her chronic lung disease, won't get much better. Has almost no family, and what she has doesn't come to see her. But I need to be more professional, not act like this."

"You mean you shouldn't get emotionally involved."

"That's right. I should carry out my duties and pat her on the shoulder and move on to the next job." She was moving her head back and forth for emphasis, eyes fixed on the floor, as if reciting a classroom dictum.

"They've got a lot of robots in Japan," I said. "Think they would work better?"

"I -- I don't know. Sometimes I wonder."

"Not me."

"Not you what, Dr. Galen?"

"I don't wonder about it. An ill patient needs a complete nurse. One with a soul. When I get sick I know who I'd want to look after me."

"Who? Who would you want, Dr. Galen?"

"You."

Linda walked over and hugged me briefly, pressing her head against my chest. It did not quite reach up to my shoulder.

"You probably wouldn't be getting a bargain," she said, mopping her eyes again.

"Neither would you, my dear," I said. "Neither would you." Then I laughed out loud.

And so did Linda.

Unprofessional? There's something worse – uncaring.

I look at the chart on the counter of the 5 North nursing station. Mrs. Theodora Atterman, age 83, had come into Dr. Fitzgibbon's office two months ago complaining of nausea and weakness. Characteristically, Dr. Fitz's dictated history and physical report is voluminous and brimming with medical and personal details. Whether she plays bridge. Whether she's as good at it as ever. Whether her family pays her enough attention. We send the medical students to read his workups: this is the way it should be done, boys and girls, the way we should all be doing it.

Mrs. A. was found to have a large, hard, nodular liver and was subsequently shown to have metastatic adenocarcinoma all over her body. Even now it is unclear what the source was. Not that it mattered -- this cancer is notoriously unresponsive to any form of therapy, including radiation or chemotherapy. Surgery, of course, was not a consideration. The patient's and family's -- and the doctor's -- decision was to keep her comfortable, and in the last week this has required hospital admission for opiate shots every three to four hours and finally a morphine drip. Everyone had agreed that when the end came no effort should be made at resuscitation. There should be "No Ward 100." She should "go in peace."

And now she has. Except that no one can die without benefit of medical supervision. Even the time of death cannot be fixed at the moment when everyone knows the patient died; it must be set at the instant when the doctor officially determines that life is absent. Legally, then, Mrs. Atterman is waiting for me.

I enter the room behind Celeste and she introduces me to the two daughters, the one son, and the daughter-in-law. Solemnly I shake their hands and move to the bedside.

The most impressive thing about Mrs. Atterman, in addition to her remarkably youthful skin and her neatly coiffed white hair, is the thing you feel about all dead persons. It's the strange stillness. It's not merely the absence of respiration that conveys the finality of this moment. Somehow you know at a glance: the life-substance has fled.

But this is not as easy as one might think. As I reach for the femoral, then the carotid, then the radial arteries, I feel a pulse! The alarum goes through my body; this must be what Eliot meant by the trilling wire in the blood. The pulse gets still stronger! And then I compose myself. This has happened many times before. I am feeling my own capillary pulse. I am a warm-hands person, and the tiny vessels in my fingers, ballooned further by the pressure of the moment, are thumping away. I listen for the heartbeat: absent. Watch for respiration: none. Test with a light for reaction of the staring pupils: no response.

But I can never "pronounce" Mrs. Atterman or, indeed, anyone, without remembering the camp.

The *camp*. I went there on an ambulance call as an intern. In that first postgraduate year, of course, we rode the ambulance everywhere it went. The driver was always a policeman and one gifted with a maniacal desire for physical danger; no call was too routine to obviate squealing tires at every turn; no assignment was too mundane to allow a speed of less than 70 through the red lights. He generally considered himself an authority on a number of points: (1) driving; (2) ambulances; (3) police methods; and of course, (4) medicine.

"What did you say this call was, Oscar?" I asked.

"Joe caught the squeal. Says 'patient not moving or breathing.'"

"Sounds like some routine pronouncing."

"Pronouncing, maybe. Routine, no."

"Why not?"

"If this is the address I heard about."

"If it is --?"

"It ain't just a house." I remember thinking at this point Oscar was having a good time.

"What, an apartment?"

"Not an apartment, either. Maybe a tent, or maybe not even a tent."

"What's this, 20 questions? Tell you what, I'll just wait and see."

Oscar was still not tired of his game. "I hear it's a camp."

I decided to keep playing for a while. "What, a camp meeting or something? Evangelistic revival? Maybe
338

somebody got too carried away, now they'll be carried away for good." I remember liking that.

"Ain't no revival, for sure. Let's see, supposed to be 369 Ashby. Here's 367, there's 371. Ain't no 369. Unless you count that alley."

"These aren't dwelling places anyway. Look like old storefronts."

"But if we go up that alley . . ." He stopped in front of the aperture between the buildings. Down that corridor, in the distance, I could see an open fire and figures moving around.

"I guess that's the camp, whatever," I said, anxious to get this over. "Let's go."

"Doc, something you oughta know."

"You mean, you're gonna break down and actually tell me what's going on?" (That was when we said "what's going on" -- before somebody invented "what's happening.")

"They say it's a gypsy camp. And you know how they are."

"No, tell me how they are."

"They believe in magic or something."

"Yes?"

"And in curses."

"Yes."

"And they don't really believe in dying."

"No?"

"So whenever a doctor says somebody's dead . . ."

"Yeah."

"They don't like it. They don't think the doctor is using his magic."

"Uh-huh."

"So they might put a curse on him --"

"I'll try to live with it."

" -- and on his family, too."

"Maybe we'll survive."

" -- Or worse."

"What's worse?"

"I don't know. Just be careful."

"Why would I worry with you here to protect me?" I remember liking that too. Sounded cool. (We were already saying "cool" then.)

On the other hand, as we started walked down the long alley, and in spite of the nippy November air, I remember not feeling particularly cool. I remember instead feeling the trilling wire in the blood that Eliot talked about. And I remember, when we arrived at the campfire and I saw the scene there, it started trilling more.

The campfire was surrounded by a circle of tents, tents of variously colored fabrics. Inside the tents and arrayed about the campfire was a semicircle of swarthy people, mostly men. Many had mustaches. Some had white or colored shirts open to the waists. A few had large knives in their belts. None had a smile on his face. All of them, men and women alike, were looking at me. Looking at my eyes. And my eyes, I realized, were blue! I couldn't remember exactly if gypsies were into evil eyes, but I did remember that evil eyes were blue.

340

I looked around for the treasure chest but saw none.

Then I looked beside the fire. An elderly woman lay in a semi-recumbent position in the arms of a strikingly beautiful dark-skinned woman with black hair. The elderly woman's jaw was slack. There was no movement in the entire area except for the flickering fire. Then the largest man in the group walked slowly toward me. He had a pleasant, sad expression on his face. He had a large, curved, not very pleasant knife in his belt. He motioned to the recumbent woman and looked at me.

"You doctor, no?"

"Yes," I said. It came out hoarse.

"You fix, yes?"

"Let me see." That came out still hoarser. I moved to the side of the elderly woman and smiled at the girl holding her head against her bosom. Her bosom was abundant and incompletely covered. The girl smiled back, briefly. I kneeled. I felt for the pulses. My capillary pulse seemed intact, clicking along at about 110 per minute. The woman's pulse was apparently absent.

The man was standing beside me. I looked up. He was huge. I felt like Jack and the beanstalk. I felt sorry for Jack having traded for those beans. And I'm sure Jack would feel sorry for me: medicine is not the only thing you can do. There's nothing really wrong with real estate.

"She's the Queen, you know," he said.

"Oh," I said.

"The Queen, you know, she cannot die."

"Oh."

There was no respiration. I listened to her heart. No sound. No carotid pulse. The pupils were dilated. The flashlight did not cause them to constrict. This particular Queen was clearly an exception to the rule about not dying.

I looked at the beautiful girl and then up at the Beanstalk Giant. "Has she been ill lately?"

"No," said the Giant.

"Was she all right today?"

"She say she feel tight in her chest," said the girl, placing her hand in the deep cleft of her own well-padded precordium. "Then she sit" (she said *seet*) "here by the fire. And then she fall over. She has not talk since then."

OK, just play it straight, Galen. Go ahead and tell them she's dead. Tell them you don't know why. Maybe she had unsuspected cancer. Maybe double pneumonia. Probably, she had a coronary and arrested. The medical examiner will probably call it natural causes and won't do a post.

Yeah, sure, see how this sounds: "I'm afraid she has passed away. The physical evidence is inadequate to establish with certainty the cause of death. Statistically coronary artery disease with an acute myocardial infarction is the most likely etiology of her sudden demise, but there are many other possibilities, and medically speaking we can't offer a conclusive statement at this time."

Great. And see how this goes: "You no good doctor. You don't even know her sickness. You fix her, you bring her back, or we fix you."

342

And how's this: the medical examiner will want to do an autopsy. On *me*. Because it won't be natural causes.

And where the hell, I thought, was Oscar. I turned and looked. He was standing in the shadows. His contribution to the proceedings seemed to be to stand at parade rest. He was not providing reassurance.

OK, I figured, at least Oscar will tell them I looked good at the last. Down in flames without a whimper. I stood. I looked off into the distance. Slowly, very slowly, I removed my stethoscope from my neck. I folded it. I placed it carefully in my pocket. I turned to the left and like a panning camera focused my eyes, evil or not, one by one into the faces of each piratical figure around the fire. Then I looked at the girl. I walked over and patted her gently on the shoulder. I turned and looked at the Beanstalk Giant. I folded my arms. I looked at the ground.

"Her heart," I said, "her great heart, has burst. It has burst in two. She has been taken away. She will not return to us in this life. There is nothing we -- you (I turned to Beanstalk) -- any of us" -- I made a sweeping, grandiloquent gesture -- "can do. Officer" --I turned to Oscar -- "call in on your police radio. They will want to confirm that no foul play has taken place. They will probably come and make an investigation. They will want to talk to me. But I will tell them that everything is all right. I will tell them that the queen has passed away of natural causes." Oscar had his pad out and seemed uncertain as to whether to write anything.

343

"I am sorry for her and for all of you," I said. "The police will come, and then you can decide about the burial." The band about the campfire seemed confused. They seemed in shock. This seemed the perfect time to leave.

"We'll wait in the street and take her away after the police come."

The police came and asked a few questions of them and one or two of me and then left – hurriedly, I thought. On the way back, with the Queen and her lovely attendant in the back, and with the trilling beginning to subside, I remember thinking that I hadn't done half bad. I remember thinking that maybe medicine was going to be all right after all.

Oscar leaned over and whispered, "Doc, you handled that pretty well. That was some bunch there, huh?"

"Another routine call, Oscar," I said. Now I was having a good time.

"But a couple of things, Doc. Why did you call the police? *I'm* the police. I could have filled out the report."

"We needed more actors on the stage, Oscar."

"Oh. And there's another thing I didn't quite catch," said Oscar.

"What's that, Oscar?"

"Exactly how did you know her heart burst?"

"Well, now, Oscar. . . "

"Yeah?"

"There are some things that only a doctor can know."

Inopportunely, the beeper goes off. I quell it by pushing a button. I turn away from the bedside to the family and simply say, "I'm sorry. I understand she was comfortable at the last."

"Yes," says one of the daughters. "She never groaned or seemed agitated. We're grateful for that. Thank you for coming."

"Certainly. I'm going to try to reach Dr. Fitz. He always wants to know."

That is an understatement. Even off call, Dr. Fitz doesn't just want to know when one of his patients expires -- he will *get livid* if you fail to call him right away.

Pulling the phone to the upper level of the nursing counter, I first write a death note on the progress sheet. Progress? We call it that. For a life of 83 years which has grieved through four major wars, official and not; watched three revolutions: cultural, sexual, and ethnic; and cheered the decline and fall of Marxism -- for all this, I say, the note I write is terribly, terribly laconic:

10/26/89 -- Called to see patient because of no vital signs. Found to have no pulse, blood pressure, respiration, pupillary reaction, or other signs of life. Pronounced dead at 1:45 a. m. ---John Galen, M. D.

I dial Fitz's home number. His wife answers.

"Hello."

"Marian, John. Is Fitz in? One of his patients expired and he always wants to hear."

"You'd better believe it. Yes, he's right here."

345

As usual, Fitz' voice is gravelly, his manner gruff. "Who is it, Mrs. Atterman?"

"Yes. She went quietly. The family's in the room. I'm getting ready to ask about a post."

"No, no, I'll talk to them."

"OK, I'll get one of the daughters to come to the phone."

"Hell no, I'll come up there. Tell them to wait. I'll be there in five minutes. Thanks."

"Whatever you say." I know there's no use arguing. Fitz is of the old school: there's no off-call when death occurs. Dr. Lewis Thomas would be interested in Fitz. That brilliant writer and teacher has pointed out that the image of the physician was better earlier in the century when his (and my) father walked the earth. Neither could do much medically but would come to just *be with* the patient and family. For this non-scientific function they were revered, even worshipped. There were no malpractice suits. Now, equipped with an imposing arsenal of drugs and techniques, we find ourselves reviled in the press and hailed before the courts. Now that we do so much, we are thought to do too little. Dr. Thomas suggests that this is a process of distancing ourselves from the patient. First, he points out, we listened with our ear against the chest -- if nothing else, a "friendly gesture." Then the stethoscope moved us back a pace. Now we send the patient across the street for a CT scan. The closeness has gone.

But Fitz will come and sit with the family and talk at length. Finally he will carry out what is surely one of the truly difficult rituals in medicine: he will ask if they want an

346

autopsy, unofficially designated a "post," for post-mortem examination. This involves opening the body cavities, removing the organs, even the brain, and examining them intently with the eye and the microscope. The reaction to this question, which unfortunately must be asked at this most tedious of all moments, is highly variable. "Oh God, no, she's suffered enough." Or, on the other hand, "Yes, we'd like to be sure about the cause of death," or even "It might help medical science."

Indeed it might, usually does. Regardless of the case and regardless of the elaborate tests and scans carried out during life, there's generally a surprise of some type to be found in the pungent arena of the autopsy lab: reactivated tuberculosis, or an unrecognized pulmonary infarction, or a deformed cardiac valve with vegetations on it. In any event, it is up to the next of kin to decide at this hard moment, and it is a question I always dread to pose.

In Mrs. Atterman's case, though, the family's response is easy to predict. They will ask Dr. Fitz what he wants to do. Does he think it will help? Is there anything he wants to know? Fitz, you see, with his gravelly voice and fake-irascible manner, has somehow managed to bypass the cold heartlessness of modern medical technology in the delicate doctor-patient-family relationship. Fitz is not across the street, Dr. Thomas. He is not distanced.

In Mrs. Atterman's room at this moment, they are electing a next of kin. It will be Fitz.

ATTACKING THE HEART ATTACK

My timing is about right as I turn the corner on 5 South: the entourage has just arrived in the Cardiac Care Unit and is just installing Henry Adams into Room 3, which is really a glassed-in-cubicle. Entourage is accurate: two nurses from the ER; a respiratory therapist, just in case; two nurses from the CCU; Dr. Wanamaker, cardiologist; Susan Pierce, his physician's assistant; and, of course, Dr. Boy. Dr. Boy, though a general internist and nephrologist like myself, has not -- or at least not yet -- relinquished the reins of this particular enterprise to the cardiologist. You can tell by the military position of his body and the frequency of his directions: "Let's put his head in first" (the nurses knew that, they do this all day); "Watch the monitor line" (one of them already had the monitor line). "Let's first transfer the top two IVs to the overhead hooks" (they knew they had to do that to get everything in the cubicle).

He was left in charge. He's still in charge. I like that.

There are now four IVs, four IV poles, an oxygen line, a cardiac monitor line, a line dangling from the BP cuff. Fortunately Henry Adams did not need an art line (intra-arterial catheter), a nasogastric tube, a Swan-Ganz monitor, a temporary pacemaker line, or a Foley catheter. It's generally assumed that the more the lines, the worse the situation, and improvement is measured by the rate at which lines can, day by day, be removed. The next time you're in the hospital, check your lines -- try to keep the number below four. Eight lines is critical indeed; ten lines is desperate. Henry at the moment is a seven-line case, primarily because of the need for inserting the four IVs ahead of time in the TPA protocol.

This substance, thromboplastin antagonist --- disrupts the clotting mechanism so thoroughly that it's not safe to stick a needle into his body anywhere after it's given -- no new IVs, no shots, no venipunctures except in places where you can put direct pressure.

We hope the stuff will dissolve the clot in his coronary artery, reestablish blood flow to the temporarily "dry" area of his cardiac muscle, prevent permanent damage, and give the cardiologists a chance to dilate up that faulty blood vessel. In the process, though, tricky things can happen. Henry may bleed somewhere, like maybe in the gastrointestinal tract; hence an ulcer patient is not a candidate. He could bleed into the brain; hence a severe hypertensive, particularly with a previous stroke, should probably be kept off the protocol. And then, if the TPA works, funny things can still take place: the newly irrigated heart muscle, now receiving its needed complement of oxygen-rich blood, may in its exuberance take on an electrical life of its own. It may become the primary pacemaker by broadcasting a fusillade of abnormal and undesirable beats. Henry must be watched like a two-year-old child playing near the street.

I walk in. Eyes flick my way momentarily to see if this interruption is acceptable. They all know me so apparently it is.

"Hi, Henry," I say. "How's it going?"

"Not too bad," he replies. Henry is being cool, too. S. I. Hayakawa in his semantics days would have called this exchange *presymbolic language*: my words and Henry's words don't exactly mean what they say. I meant, "I'm here,

349

Henry. I care about you." Henry meant, "I know you're there. I'm determined to do my part, though I'm not so foolish as to pretend that this is a picnic." Sometimes it's good to have a code.

"Any change in the cardiogram yet?" I ask.

Dr. Boy holds up a strip. "Let me just show you what happens when you call in a real pro." It's clear Dr. Boy has acquired the doctor's rhetoric: claim credit when things go right; when things go wrong, blame nature.

The ST elevation has reverted essentially to normal:

Before TPA

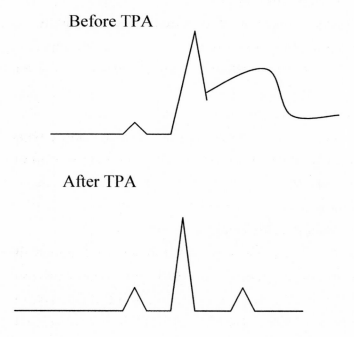

After TPA

"Great. Any arrhythmias?"

"Funny you should ask," says Paul Wanamaker. "He had a lot of coupling. We started him on a lidocaine drip.

Then he had a couple of blasts of v. tach. Terminated them with lidocaine boluses. We've been thinking about Norpace or more beta-blockers but we've held off, going mainly with the Xylocaine. Pretty typical reperfusion behavior so far." This last is not so much to educate me, in case I'm not *au courant*, as is it is to establish the expertise of Dr. Wanamaker, in case I was not already aware of it.

"Think you'll take a look at his arteries, when, 36 hours or so?"

"No, in about 6 hours. Push ahead earlier if EKG changes come back or pain reappears."

"Henry, looks like you're in good hands, my friend."

"I can tell, Doctor, I can tell."

I look at Wanamaker and then Dr. Boy. "I'll be around."

"So will we," says Dr. Boy.

I walk outside the cubicle and nod at Lora and Gwen who are sitting at the big monitor desk. "Keep up the good work," I offer.

"Dr. Galen, don't we always?"

"As a matter of fact, yes."

I reach the elevators and ponder whether to check in the operating room or start the paperwork. The decision proves easy: I punch the first floor, where the OR is. While the elevator makes up its mind, buzzes, and slowly closes its door, I think back to the old days of treating coronaries.

Old days? Only thirty years ago a heart attack was brought in and put in bed. Maybe give him oxygen, decide whether to give anticoagulants. Give him digitalis if there was any sign of failure. There were no monitors. If he had a rhythm upset, too bad, maybe the nurse would catch it on her next round. If he had cardiac arrest, that was too bad, too: either let him go or open the chest and squeeze the heart directly -- we didn't know about closed cardiac compression. We didn't intubate people on the floor. Lidocaine drips were unknown. There were no beta blockers, no TPA, no Norpace, no calcium-channel blockers. There was no coronary angiography, no balloon angioplasty, no stents, no lasers, no pacemakers, no coronary artery bypass surgery. Now we work on them, get them fixed up, get them out of bed, send them home in a week even if they have open-heart surgery, start an exercise program in a few weeks. Then they stayed in bed three weeks, went home to a limited life. If they weren't sick when they came in, they were when they left. Progress is our most important product. *Our?* *Their* (the gutsy researchists who did all this). And then sometimes we don't make progress, we go backwards. Ask Fitz or Lewis Thomas.

ATTENTION -- WARD 100 -- CCU. ATTENTION -- WARD 100 -- CCU.

Jesus Christ. Henry Adams.

As previously noted, you don't use the elevator when a Ward 100 erupts: you revert to more primal behavior and run up the steps. Back in CCU I find Henry's room is jammed with people.

"What happened, Lora?"

"V. tach, degenerating into v. fib. They're shocking him now."

352

Ventricular tachycardia: abnormal rhythm originating from an outlaw focus low down in the cardiac architecture. Not a good rhythm because, number one, it's fast -- maybe 160 a minute -- but also not good because, number two, it's not very effective. The blood pressure may drop or the heart itself may go into failure.

But number *three* and worst of all, this aberrant type of beat may herald the dreaded ventricular fibrillation -- a totally ineffective state of electrical chaos, equivalent to cardiac arrest. And that's happening to Henry Adams now. I decide not to enter Henry's cubicle because: (1) there's nothing I could add; (2) I don't want to get in the way; and (3) I couldn't physically get in there anyway. But there is something I can do out here:

Lord, let the defibrillating current work and revert him to a normal rhythm. Please don't make them have to resuscitate him, press on his chest, break some ribs. With that TPA he could bleed into his chest, maybe his pericardium. Please make him revert. Please.

There is a sudden relaxation of shoulders in the crowded room. Doctor Boy turns around.

"Back in normal sinus. Think we'll go with an osmolol drip. We've had enough of this, right Dr. Wanamaker?"

"Right."

Forever cool, we doctors. Except when we have to call on higher authority. Then we get kind of humble. But as I head back toward the operating room, riding the senescent

353

elevator, it hits me with a jolt: even in my most abject appeal I managed to be patronizing.

I explained TPA to the Lord!

SANCTUM, SANCTORUM

The Operating Room -- not a room at all but a suite of about 30 rooms -- is strategically designed to intimidate the non-surgeon. To begin with, there are signs all over the place forbidding trespass:

DO NOT ENTER. AUTHORIZED PERSONNEL ONLY. DO NOT USE AS A PASSAGEWAY.

These signs convey the unstated but unequivocal implication that non-procedural, merely cognitive, people like internists are *personna non grata.* Probably inherently contaminated.

But the signs are fairly subtle compared to the Red Line.

The Red Line extends across the corridor as it branches off to the active surgical area. It is about eight inches wide. It is not merely red, it is Chinese red. Its mute crimson says: Do not cross me unless you are fully attired in sacred garb, with that little toy cap on your head, the suffocating little mask on your face, the pajama-like scrub suit on your body, and those impossible elasticized paper sacks over your shoes. Presumably you have crossed yourself upon reaching this Hall of Halsted, this Lair of Lister. This

354

holy place is not for just anyone. Hast thou made thyself pure?

If one is jaded, like me, and if it's the wee hours, one finds it within oneself to eschew such choreography. In other words, I go to the intercom and press Room 9, where Barton is working on Egbert. Even, so, as the static comes on, I do have just the slightest sensation of calling into the chapel and interrupting the high priests as they labor over their shrine.

"Earl? Galen. How's it coming?"

"Fine. She's doing well. Looks like you were right."
"Right? Hell, all I knew, she needed a surgeon."
"Yeah, but I mean about the appendix."
"What about it?"
"You said it was too perfect."
"Uh-oh. What is it, then?"
"A Meckel's. With pancreatic tissue. And bleeding into the sac. Good thing we operated. The appendix is normal. 'Course we'll get that out too while we're here." Earl had found a congenital outpouching, or diverticulum, with glandular tissue which was releasing digestive enzymes.

"Great, Earl. Anything I can contribute?"
"No, sir. Just find us some more of these."
"See what I can do."

A Chance to Cut is a Chance to Cure. It's the name of a book. Written by a young surgeon.

NO MORE ASPIRIN

Mary Lewis is sitting up in the chair in her bedside cubicle in ICU Blue, smiling.

"You're beginning to look pretty sassy, young lady," I suggest.

"I'd be moreso if they'd let me have a cigarette."

"Doesn't go with the decor down here. Or the oxygen, either."

"But I love the gown. Now *it* goes with anything." Mary holds out the cotton fabric which swathes her. It has a tiny blue pattern, maybe little butterflies on a beige background, with the words PROPERTY OF METRO NORTH HOSPITAL in black letters near the hem. (Sometimes they get garments from *another* hospital, in which case the words are PROPERTY OF SOUTH MADISON COUNTY HOSPITAL. They use the gowns anyway.) It has ties in the back which are just beyond the reach of even a perfectly well person; thus the garment does not discriminate against the handicapped -- nobody can fasten it without help.

"Those are gotten up special for us by SACKS Fifth Avenue. That's S-A-C-K-S."

"Guess it's appropriate for a bag like me."

"Wouldn't say that. Matter of fact, you're beginning to shape up now. How'd you like to get out of here -- out of ICU, that is. Go to a private room. It'll be quieter."

"Great. Do I take my friend here with me?" She motions to the IV pole with its translucent bag of fluid.

"Just for tonight. Your blood work looks almost normal now. The acid-base balance studies are back to

356

normal.   You dodged a bullet, you understand that, don't you?"

"Now I know.   When they say take two aspirin and call me in the morning --"

"Yes?"

"I guess they don't mean every two hours."

VIS-A-VIS

"Did Dr. Brandt see you, Rhonda?   You know, the psychiatrist?"

"Oh, yes."   Rhonda is dwarfed by the geri-chair in which she is sitting next to her ICU bed.   She smiles broadly but not without a little sardonic curl to her left lower lip.   Her teeth are in good repair.   They need to be, what with the Vassar clench.   "We had a simply delightful little *tete-a-tete*."

"I think that means head-to-head, so did you?   I mean, get your heads together?"

"In a way.   He thinks I need to go to the funny farm, Dr. Galen.   Me!   Off to the laughing academy!"

"That's what they usually think when somebody tries to shuffle off the old mortal coil.   They figure there's a need for attitude adjustment.   And not something a couple of martinis can fix."

"So --"   now in imperious mode -- "I guess I'll go to the unit here.   It's good, isn't it?"

"It's my choice locally.   Not that it's exactly a spa.   Dr. Brandt can supervise things there.   What about that, Rhonda?   Are you two -- do you seem to be -- *sympatico*?"   That seemed like a good Vassar/Smith word.

357

"Oh, yes, he's perceptive and . . . knowing."

"Good. Maybe you can be transferred directly in the morning."

"John --"

"Yes, Rhonda."

"You'll -- I mean, see me there too?"

"Sure. Keep up with your wiring and plumbing and so forth."

"And also my -- I mean, you're not going to give up on me." Here *up* is the operative word, pronounced *op* and ejected into the room with a prominent jaw-jut.

"Not now, for God's sake. I've done all the hard work on you. Now I need to get some credit."

BESSIE REVISITED

Bessie Sinclair looks less puffy than this morning. Her oxygen cannula has slipped down around her neck but she doesn't seem in any respiratory distress.

"How'd you like that washing machine, Miss Bessie?"

"Not bad, Doc. Seems like I've got more room to breathe or something." She raises her arms and inhales, as if to demonstrate.

"Sure -- that kidney machine pulled some of that excess fluid out. Let's see, you lost, what" -- I open the chart and flip to the dialysis record -- "seven pounds." This one sheet is loaded with data -- time on machine, time off, pre- and post- weight in kilograms, serial blood pressures, heparin doses, description of kidney type, etc.

I listen to her chest. Rales still. Fluid still there but less than this morning.

"Coming along, Bessie. We keep this up, you'll make the Olympics."

"Watch them on TV, you mean."

"Guess that's more realistic. . . for you and me both."

"That's plumb good enough for me."

Those ills we have. Bessie is dealing with them.

ENCORE, SATCHMO

Thomas Hopper has a broad smile too but there's no sardonic twist like Rhonda. Satchmo doesn't have a sardonic twist in his entire soul.

"I think Dr. Boy done fixed me up."

"He been checking on you, Thomas?"

"Just like mother love."

I run through a survey neuro exam. Nothing new. Nothing to suggest swelling of his brain or expansion of the blood clot in Thomas' head. His heart, though, is "tacking" -- speeding -- along as usual. His gallop -- signifying heart failure -- is present as always. With Thomas we don't have much room to maneuver .

"Does this mean I can quit worrying about you, Thomas?"

"Nawsir, Doc. I don't never want you to quit worrying. But maybe sometimes you and Dr. Boy can take turns."

SCRUBS

I see Dr. Johnathan Minter down the hall, coming my way. Johnathan's standard gait, like that of all cardiovascular-thoracic surgeons (i. e., The Super-Chosen) is at least a swagger. He socks his knuckles against the wall rail as he goes, not so much (one senses) to orient himself as to stabilize the wall, to infuse the inanimate world about him with a mote or two of his intrinsic power.

Under his long white lab coat he is wearing flimsy cotton tops and pants officially known in the trade as "scrubs." These are what you put on when you get ready to do an operation. Scrubs are thus the talisman of the proceduralist -- the surgeons, the cardiac cath doctors, the radiologists who run catheters and drains into patients. I used to wear them sometimes when putting a patient on the artificial kidney, before the engineers improved the device and before the technicians took over. Now it's the technicians who wear the scrubs. Nurses wear blue scrubs, red scrubs, yellow scrubs depending one which unit they work in, except that they don't utter the names of primary colors but call them aquamarine, hot pink, and canary. Regular civilians like to get hold of scrubs and lounge in them, work in the yard in them, sleep in them.

For, you see, scrubs resemble nothing so much as a pair of pajamas. I've often wondered if the surgeons each morning change directly from their pajamas into scrubs, and then back again. Sleep in pajamas, work in scrubs? Or maybe change from day scrubs into night scrubs. Or maybe even not change -- just wear the same set for 24 hours.

What is clear is that scrubs identify you as a *doer*, someone who does things to people, and so scrubs are worn as a shibboleth of your special gifts. They are your badge. *Sartor Resartus*, said Carlyle. Clothes make the man.

"Think we got Mrs. Whatsaname fixed up, John. Lady with the unstable pacer." They, The SuperChosen, never know patients' names. So many, you know. So many supplicants for the magic.

"Mrs. Croft," I offer. I must keep up with the names, you see, being hopelessly unchosen and therefore bereft of occult powers. "Great, Johnny. See this very often? I mean, pacer flopping around like that, causing it to malfunction?" *Translation: I've never heard of this happening before but in case it's common I don't want to look uncool.*

"Yeah, well, some of them do flop around in the pocket. I think this was the first one that we've actually seen lose contact. (*We.*) One of the connection points was loose when we got in there. Interesting case. She's in, let's see, where is Mrs. Whatsaname, Jane?" The SC never know room numbers, either.

Jane, the physician's assistant (PA) walks up. "She's in 341, Dr. Minter. How are you, Dr. Galen?" A very attractive strawberry blonde with no makeup, wearing a long white coat over a tiny-figured silk pantsuit, Jane rewards me with a brilliant smile. The smile, however, is brief.

"Good, Jane. You folks been busy?"

"We try to keep him" -- she motions to Johnathan -- "moving along."

"Well, thanks to both of you for curing Mrs. Croft. When can she go home, do you think?"

"Tomorrow, if the pacer behaves," says Johnathan. "Think Mark is going to move her around in the morning, get her to raise her arms and so forth while she's on telemetry. She should do well."

Now that she's had the magic.

Dr. Minter is wearing *red* scrubs, sure sign of the cardiac surgery unit. He walks off down the main corridor, Jane in tow, knocking his knuckles against the wall.

FOG BREAKING

I walk into Harold Patton's room. He looks pretty good. He is smiling. He doesn't seem confused at all now. The Mrs. is sitting in the corner, trying to hide her cigarette.

"Did the pharmacist ever call, Mrs. Patton?"

"Oh, yes, she called and talked to Harold."

"Was she still crying?"

"Yes, I think she was."

"What did she say?"

"Well, she said how sorry she was, and asked how he was doing, and wanted to know if she could do anything. Harold said no. But she said she wanted to do something anyway."

"What did she do?"

"She put the drug store manager on the line, " says Harold.

"What did he say?"

"Said he was going to give me a full refund on the medicine they fouled up on."

LIFE, DEATH OR WHAT?

Jeffrey Owens, MD, is walking down the hall toward me. Strands of brunette hair are hanging in his face. He looks tired.

"How'd the conference go with Sydney's family, Jeffrey?"

"OK, I guess. They said they couldn't stand to see him suffer, they wanted to let him out of his misery. I told them he didn't know what was happening, probably wouldn't remember anything. I said he has a fair-to-middlin' chance of complete recovery. Then I thought about our conversation, and decided I should be a little more definite here."

"What'd you say?"

"I told them that I wanted to give him a full-court press, that I didn't think it would be medically or legally right to stop support measures. Then I said that if they wanted to stop trying they would have to put another doctor in charge. Then I left them to think it over."

"What finally happened?"

"They said they wanted me to push ahead, give him every chance. That made me feel better. Then they said something that reassured me even more."

"What was that, Jeffrey?"

"They said they didn't want another doctor."

PLASTICS, PLASTICS!

I pick up Rufus Conway's chart in ICU Blue and turn to "Doctors' Progress Notes." After all, I'm on call and might get paged to make decisions about him. I'd need to be familiar with what happened, wouldn't I?

OK, so I'm curious as hell about the guy we scooped up off the floor.

The newest entry is by Dr. Jardin, vascular surgeon. One of my patients, a graphologist, has taught me a few of the essentials of handwriting analysis (and then partly allayed my skepticism by accurately describing all the personalities in our office from their writing). Now I apply my new-found analytical ability to Dr. Jardin's script. Let's see: upright characters, slight right lean, upward trend of the baseline, no looping at the top, *t*'s crossed firmly in the upper half of the stem. Interpretation: strong ego structure, rarely reliant on others, successful, confident, unafraid.

Nailed. Maybe graphology isn't such a fringe science after all.

Brief Op Note

Preop dx -- rupt abd aortic aneurysm

Postop dx -- same

Pathol -- 6 x 10 cm. aneurysm extending from below renals to bifurcation, sl aneurysmal change R iliac. 2 cm.

364

perforation posteriorly. Peri-
aortic hematoma est. 700 ml.
  <u>Procedure</u> -- Y graft as
shown. Dacron # K301365
Yurushi Pharm.
  <u>Post Op Status</u>: Stable.
EBL -- 5000 ml. Replaced with 8
units PK cells, 7 L D-5-RL.

  EBL -- Estimated Blood Loss -- 5000 milliliters -- 5 liters -- 5 1/2 quarts! All the blood in a small person's body! Replaced with red blood cells and then another 7 liters -- 8 quarts -- of fluid. Where did it all go? The final entry says:

Pt. tol. well. To RR in good condition.

  Patient tolerated the procedure well? Sent to the Recovery Room in good condition?

  Yep. Just like that.

  Earlier, checking on Rufus, a shadow had fallen over the page. I looked around. It had been Elbert Williams, here to check on Rufus. Towering over me, the chart, everything. Casting shadows on the chart. Casting shadows everywhere.

  "Did great," he said..

  "Yeah. Funny he was in such profound shock, only lost 700 cc. To begin with"

  "I noticed that."

  "Maybe the expanding blood collection caused a vasovagal reaction."

"Yeah. Or something. Had a slow pulse in the office."

"Well, good work, y'all," I said at the time. "Good thing he didn't get caught in traffic. Even after he got here he had a 50 % mortality."

"Not with this team," says Elbert.

"How do you mean?"

"Not with four on the floor."

JIMMY'S NEW MACHINE

Jimmy Treadway is now on dialysis; that is, blood is coming out of one channel of the tube positioned below his right clavicle and is flowing in the other.

And things are not going all that well with Jimmy.

"Can't get decent flow, eh, Eileen?"

"Nossir, any time we get above 150 ml/min his pressure drops out."

"How about some mannitol?"

"Did that already."

"How about albumin?"

"Could do that."

"Let's."

Jimmy is coming and going mentally, but he has to be sedated so he won't fight the ventilator.

"What do we think about his mental status?"

From the other side of the bed Jennifer answers. "Oh, let that Versed wear off and he's a tiger. Also non-contrast head CT was reported as normal."

366

"Good. How about cardiac indices?" I can't just restrict myself to the kidneys.

"Well, they decided not to put in a Swan, thought it would just add problems," Jennifer says. "His CVP is kicking around 4-8."

"That may be a little low. Ask Dr. Middleton if we can't push volume a little – fluid or more blood."

"He said go ahead with another two units of packed cells if the CVP stays below 6."

"Good."

"Dr Galen? Can I ask a question?"

"Sure, Jennifer."

"Do you think his kidneys can recover? He's so young and all."

"Definitely. If we get everything else under control, his kidneys can get back to normal."

"How long do you think that might be?"

"Depends on a lot of things. If his blood pressure stays unstable, the kidney failure could go on indefinitely. If we get him on a plateau, he should recover much more promptly."

"You mean, like a couple of days?"

"I mean, like a couple of weeks."

"How can we get him through that?"

"By doing what we're doing – arranging for him to have a date with Eileen about every day."

DOCUMENTATION

You can be sure it hasn't gone away; at 2:15 a. m. it's still waiting.

The paperwork.

It's easy to put off while you take care of the patients. In fact, how can you even justify leaving a sick person's bedside to generate a paper trail? But just collapse in bed and let it go, you've got all kinds of trouble. The medical records people call your secretary and send you messages. They use terms you haven't heard since high school, like incomplete, tardy, delinquent. Your secretary worries; you even worry that maybe you aren't her hero any more. The medical records librarians all recognize you, they give you a knowing look in the hall. They turn to each other. They're probably saying "I think he's one of them."

The Medical Records Committee, consisting of other doctors and some of the administrative people, writes you truly insulting letters. They suggest that, since you surely know the importance of full and timely documentation, your tardiness clearly brands you as a medical outlaw. They indicate that they are about to invoke the rule which throws you off the staff. You may have failed to dictate a discharge summary or two (or twelve). Or you may have -- horror of horrors -- left off the signature on a "May Go" order or even left blank one of the signature boxes on the ER. (Twenty years ago there was one box and last year there were four boxes. This may be a trend.)

Then they post The List. The List is a littany of the Untouchables, the doctors who, *ugh,* have overdue charts. It is placed in plain view in the Record Room and other places.

You get your own personal copy through interoffice mail. It is designed to invoke Peer Pressure. It is the modern equivalent of The Stocks. It is, apparently, the ultimate punishment.

People who are on the Medical Records Committee get there largely through no fault of their own -- they are appointed by the Medical Staff Executive Committee. They have no unique status or training and their own records are not necessarily examples of Modern Literature. On the other hand, they have not done anything wrong, either. In other words, they are regular folks.

But the Chairman of the Medical Record Committee is something special. He is one of the top three or four obsessive-compulsive people on the staff. His histories and consultations are endless, performed within minutes, dictated with elaborate articulation (including grimaces as he speaks into the machine), dated correctly, and signed promptly, even if, truth be told, they are not always Deathless Prose. He has never personally been on The List, of course, and seems to have a slightly different manner when he speaks to those who are. He unquestionably sat up front in Social Studies. There have been several such Chairmen during my time, and I have always pictured them in the entrails of the Record Room signing the Bad Letter with expressions of glee. Their preoccupation with paper, I have always suspected, probably extends beyond the record department – perhaps to the restroom: I would bet on consumption of about one-half roll per day.

But, let's face it, documentation is essential. You must put down accurate observations, or they are of no value. You must do it at the time, or you forget. Someone coming after should be able to read what you wrote and understand it, to get some idea of your thinking. Without this, there is no way to carry out good continuous care, no way to defend yourself or the hospital in court, no way for your colleagues to carry out quality evaluation. Most of all, without good records, clinical studies can't be done to find out the best way to treat patients in the future. In other words, without a good paper trail, medical progress is impossible.

So I make paper rounds at 2:20 a. m. One by one, I go to the chart racks of each new patient in the nursing stations and dictate a history and physical examination. In the complicated case of Randolph Brown, the kidney patient with the high potassium, it will run to three single-spaced typewritten pages. The nurses' notes are lengthier -- 4 1/2 pages are included, full of notations like:

10:05 p. m. -- BP 100 systolic (Doppler). P 61 R 24. Skin pale. Alert. Rhythm sinus bradycardia. Seems in moderate distress. IV dripping at 50 ml/min as ordered. ~
10:06 p. m. -- Ca gluconate, one amp (900 mgm) IV per cathlon -- verbal order Dr. J. G.

And on and on, minute by minute. We could never run the show without good nurses. Good meaning competent. And competent meaning perfectionistic. It is important to have a good medical staff and good hospital administration, but that's primarily because they attract fine nurses, the heart and soul of any medical operation.

The abdominal pain of Mrs. Egbert is covered more succinctly.

CHIEF COMPLAINT: "My stomach hurts"

PRESENT ILLNESS: This 36-year-old Caucasian female was well until approximately 10 p. m. on the night prior to admission, at which time she observed the onset of a vague sense of abdominal disquiet. By midnight she had a slight epigastric ache. She slept fitfully and awoke the next morning with no appetite and generalized upper abdominal distress. She ate no breakfast and only a few crackers for lunch along with a few sips of milk. At about 1 p. m. she vomited once, approximately one cupful of ingested material with yellow staining, no blood. By 5 p. m. her discomfort had migrated to the RLQ and became progressively more intense. She noted that local pressure caused pain and that jarring as by walking caused exacerbation of the localized pain. She arrived at the ER on my instructions at about 11 p. m. She had one small BM about 10 a. m. on the day of admission.

PAST HISTORY: Usual childhood diseases without complication or sequelae. Scarlet fever age 3 without known residue. Tonsillectomy-adenectomy age 5. D& C 1987 for menometrorrhagia -- benign results.

FAMILY HISTORY: Maternal grandmother with late-onset diabetes mellitus, alive and well. Paternal uncle with hypertension and cornonary disease. Not other serious familial diseases.

SOCIAL HISTORY: Works part-time at local Mission Board. Lives with husband. Childless.

PERSONAL HISTORY: Does not drink alcoholic beverages. Never smoked. No regular medications. Occasional aspirin, antihistamine.

371

REVIEW OF SYSTEMS: ENT: Occ hay fever. No sinusitis. CARDIORESP: No dyspnea, orthopnea, chest pain, hypertension, asthma, recent respiratory infection. GI: Rare indigestion and heartburn. Otherwise neg. except as in Present Illness. GU: No dysuria, urgency, nocturia, flank pain, chills or fever. GYN: LMP as noted 2 weeks ago. No pregnancies. Last pelvic 8 months ago -neg. NEURO: Neg. ORTH: Not remarkable.

PHYSICAL EXAMINATION: T 100 F. P 88 R 18 BP 100/62
SKIN: Pink without cyanosis.
Details of the exam are described as normal except:
.ABDOMEN:
Flat.   Generally soft without tenderness to light palpation except in RLQ, where there is exquisite tenderness and marked guarding. There is also rebound tenderness, rebound referral, and positive psoas sign. Bowel sounds slightly hypoactive.
RLQ pain on jarring when patient stands on toes
*   and then and drops to heels.*
ASSESSMENT: Acute appendicitis until proved otherwise. Consider but doubt: ectopic pregnancy, endometriosis, ruptured ovarian cyst, Crohn's disease, etc.

*   PLAN: CBC, SMA-18, amylase, pregnancy test, ua, surgical consultation. IV fluids. Abd films and/or gastrograffin enema only if desired by surgeon. Expect RLQ exploration required.. NEUROLOGICAL: Mental status, cranial nerves, cerebellar function, sensory*

Now the writing of the History and Physical reveals little narrative talent. It is replete with jargon, abbreviations, medical slang, and pedantry, but that's the way we do it. You could translate it into simple English a la Strunk & White, convert it into Elizabethan style with a Shakespearean flourish, or make it Hemingway-esque with taut monosyllables -- and any of the three would probably be clearer and more graceful. But then you would be *declasse* in the Record Room, and God knows, we wouldn't want to be that, there.

So let it be. Sorry, E. B., Will, Papa.

My surgeon-tennis-partner Dr. Frank Wharton maintains that the length of a consultation is inversely proportional to its value. That is, a two- or three-page report indicates that the writer has no clue what's wrong; a two- or three-line notation reflects great confidence. There may be some truth in this.

I can remember one of my mentors' scoring solidly in this category. Asked to evaluate the patient's enlarged heart, this great cardiologist and clinician was able to determine from bedside evaluation that she had low thyroid function, causing fluid in the sac around the heart -- making it appear large -- as well as a multitude of other symptoms. Treatment of this condition, everybody knew, is simple. His consultation was laconic:

> *Dx.: Myxedema*
>
> *Rx.: Synthroid*
>
> *--RBL*

I've gone this far, might as well check by the Record Room to make sure I don't have any incomplete charts which might surface into the dreaded delinquent classification.

While I'm there I can stop by the Record Room bathroom.

See if there's any paper left.

PERCHANCE TO DREAM

"Josie, what would happen if I stretched out on the bed in 6 for a few minutes? Would I get reported to housekeeping? I'm waiting on a few people to get a little better before I go home." *But not necessarily before I sleep.*

"No sir," says Josie. I'll promise you won't get in any trouble whatsoever. I'm running this place now, you know."

"I knew that. I got the report that you were the charge nurse in ICU Blue. Congratulations. They're lucky to have somebody like you."

"Thank you, sir."

Josie is an extremely neat and extremely intelligent black woman about 35 who started out as a ward clerk years ago. She was so quick and so talented with patients that several of us encouraged her to enter nursing school. She did and led her class all the way to her baccalaureate degree. Then she went from nurse-intern to floor nurse, then unit charge nurse, then took advanced ICU training.

Last month she was offered a unit director's job -- that is, the administrative management of two nursing stations – but she declined, saying she wanted to nurse people, not a clipboard. Then the ICU head nurse got pregnant, and here Josie is, continuing her usual superlative ways.

"I've left word with the operator where I am and I've also got the beeper."

"We'll call you if they need you. You rest, Dr. Galen."

I lie down on the firm hospital bed, put my hands behind my head, and look at my watch: 3:08. Four seconds later I get two beeps, but my watch now says 3:53. Funny how my watch and I disagree sometimes.

374

"Randolph's K+ is 5.9 now."

"Great."

"When do you want another one?"

"About 5 a. m."

"Call you?"

"Only if it's above 6 or below 4. . . ."

DEAD RINGER

"Doctor, this is Carl, with LifeLink. You taking care of a female named Coberly, K. G.?"   The voice on the line sounds automatic.

"K. G.? Is that Karen Coberley?"

"Let me look. Karen G. Coberley. Date of birth, 3/26/60."

"Yeah. Name's right. DOB's about right. That's her. What's up?"

"A kidney. Three-antigen match. Almost like an identical twin."

"Dear God."

"Is she is in shape for transplant? I mean, before we call her."

"Sure.   Great. I saw her today, I mean yesterday. Some fistula trouble, but she'll be thrilled out of her mind."

"Fine.   We'll try her at home.   We have her number and she also has a beeper."

"Wonderful."

"Thanks, Doctor."

"OK. No, hey, wait! *Carl!*"

"Yessir."

"She's *here*! I mean in the damn hospital. Had her fistula fixed."

"At North Metro?"

"Right."

"Very good. Dr. Henderson will do her there, I'm sure. Do you know her room number?"

"It's 416."

"Of course we'll have to do a cross-match with the donor blood."

"Sure."

"I'll call her right now."

"No, don't."

"Sir?"

"Don't call her."

"Pardon?"

"I'm going up there right now. *Then* you call her."

Karen is sleeping peacefully. Her head is half-submerged under the pillow, her short, coal-black hair trailing from under the pillow-slip.

"Karen."

No response.

"Karen." Louder.

She stirs slightly. I touch her shoulder. She extends both arms and stretches. Then she turns my way.

"Dr. Galen . What in the world time is it?"

"It's late. I mean early.   Karen, wake up, I need to talk to you."

"What is it?"

"Some great news, but I don't want you to get too excited yet."

She sits bolt upright and flips both legs off the side of the bed. Her eyes are enormous. "Tell me -- quick!"

"They have a kidney for you. But --"

She jumps out of bed and hugs me. And hugs. And doesn't let go. I hug back, of course. Here I am, in a woman's bedroom, a patient, I'm the doctor, she's in her nightgown, we're hugging. This would never pass inspection by the compliance officer. *Doctors never touch patients except to shake hands or examine them.* Sure, except maybe three or four times a day: something good happens in the doctor-patient relationship and we hug. Sometimes men and men. Please don't tell the compliance officer.

"But -- Karen, we've got to do a cross-match, of course. It'll probably be all right, but there's always a chance of things not working out."

"Oh, I know, I know, I could be incompatible. But I won't. I *feel* it."

"They'll be coming to draw the blood now. Karen --"
"Yes, sir?"

"If everything's OK, this kidney is a nearly perfect match."

"Terrific! You mean, maybe a two-antigen match?"
"Three."

"Oh, my God. All that hoping and praying, then --"
"Yes."

As I turn to go, the lab technologist comes into Room 416 with her blood-drawing tray.

The hoping and praying aren't over.

CALL TO ARMS

Joy and triumph have not always been the rule with the kidney transplantation saga. Before 1966 there was no such thing; patients of all ages gradually went downhill and died from kidney failure. Their doctors, like yours truly, just watched them. Then, in Seattle, they developed chronic dialysis. And then, beginning in Boston and later in Richmond, Virginia, successful transplantation of a relative's kidney, or even a cadaver organ, became possible. We started at Jones Medical Center in late 1966. The first one was a hospital-wide enterprise: the nurses, the clerks, the orderlies were all involved and cheering. This initial effort and the second one were both eventual failures. But as techniques, drugs, cross-matching, and luck got better, the success rate rose from 40% to 60% and finally, now, to 85%. A good transplanted kidney returns a very sick person almost to normal health, more so than chronic dialysis.

But the early days were strenuous. We had no funds; not until 1972 did Congress provide coverage through Medicare. Prominent citizens in the patient's home town had to start fund-raising drives. They sponsored fun runs, fish fries, parades to pay the huge expense of hospitalization for donor and recipient, the surgery, the medication.

I will surely never forget The Call. The overhead page said to contact the Chief Administrator's office.

"John, can you come down right away? There's someone here I'd like you to talk to," said Boswell Hanover.

Boswell and I had had a few run-ins of a minor degree. But I said, Sure.

When I knocked on the ornate door of the Chief Adminstrative Suite and entered, there was no way I could have been prepared for what greeted me.

The Klieg lights hit me in the eyes so strongly I couldn't see the person in front of me, but I *could* see the microphone which was thrust into my face.

"Dr. Galen, why are you letting this woman die?" said a female voice.

"What woman?" was my brilliant retort.

"Mrs. Andrus, Janie Andrus."

I now recognized the speaker as Ellen Karlton, a rather notorious local TV investigative reporter. But I wasn't going to let her off that easily.

"Another question – Who are *you*?"

"You must know – Ellen Karlton, reporter for WCHO-TV."

I wasn't going to cave in. Also I needed time to think.

"Still another question – why are you here? Why have you set up what looks like a studio in the Administrator's office?"

"We want to know why this patient is being denied a kidney transplant."

"Well, she isn't being *denied* anything. She's getting all the care that modern medicine can provide. I really should tell you some things. How much time do you have?"

"Not all day, Dr. Galen. We just want the facts."

"Good. The facts will take 90 seconds. Do you have 90 seconds?"

"Yes." Ellen seemed about to fume.

"First, do you have a written release from the patient for me to talk to you?"

"Of course not, Doctor. We're the *Press*, for God's sake."

"All the more reason to have a release. But I'll bypass that under the circumstances. The patient in kidney failure can be helped by a kidney transplant if three conditions are met. One, she would need a donor. Two, she would need some source of funds. Three, the patient must have a condition which can be helped by a transplant.

This lady *has* a donor—her brother. She and her family don't have private sources, but the banker in Ackerville has just told me they have raised forty thousand dollars—more than enough. But the patient has systemic inflammation of all the blood vessels in her body. A transplant wouldn't help that. She is in no condition for any kind of surgery. So she has two out of three requirements, but the most important thing she doesn't have – the ability to respond to treatment. Any further questions?" I glance at my watch.

"Yes, Doctor. How much are you charging her?"

I pull a little notebook out of my pocket and pretend to consult it. It's actually blank.

Then I look up at Ellen. "Nothing," I respond.

"And why is that, Doctor?"

"I thought you understood. She has no funds."

No story from Ellen Karlton appeared on the six- or eleven o'clock news that night.

From that point on, I recall, there was a trend toward improvement in the transplant PR situation.

HYPERVENTILATION, OR...?

I wake, finally in my own bed, staring at the ceiling wondering what that noise is. It's not the normal phone, it's not the beeper. Am I on call? Oh yes -- it's that *new* phone, the electronic one with the undefinable whimper. I turn the light on and pick up the instrument. It's 4:21 a. m. by the digital clock, but I am of course awake, composed, in charge.

"Hello." My voice cracks.

"Dr. Galen, this is the answering service. Telephone call from Dr. Williams' patient. Mrs Ellen Sievert. Shortness of breath. 873-9933."

"Thanks." I try to remember the number as a matter of self-discipline. Also I can't find a pencil.

I dial, the phone rings, then it starts that beep-beep-beep, and the lady with the lovely voice comes on and is just absolutely delighted to tell me there is no such number in the 404 area. How can she be so thrilled to tell me that? Her voice sounds exactly as if, during this phone conversation, someone she really likes is tickling her in an erogenous area. Employee benefits at the telephone company are getting out of hand. And on duty, after midnight, too.

I try dialing again. Same results. The lady tells me the same thing, in the same euphoric tone. Her hedonistic pursuits seem to be progressing nicely. I call the answering service back, wait while they dig up the number on the computer. It's 873-*9993*. Maybe I should get a pencil. I dial. It's busy. Shall I declare an emergency at 4:22 am? I grab my glasses, find the redial button and keep pressing it. Finally I get through.

"Oh, hello, Dr. Williams."

"Dr. Galen."

"Who?"

"Dr. Galen. I'm Dr. Williams' partner. I'm on call for him tonight, er, this morning. Also, I think we met in the office one day, Mrs. Sievert."

"Oh, yes, Dr. Galen, you've got that cute grand-daughter. She was up there one day. And call me Helen."

"Thanks, Helen. Now what seems to be bothering you?"

"I'm so short of breath. It just won't go down all the way. And I'm so lightheaded, like I'm going to pass out or float away or something. My hands and feet are, you know, like numb and tingling at the same time? Can they be? And every once in a while my fingers draw up, you know, like in a claw. What's happening, am I having a heart attack? Am I dying?"

"I don't think so, not at all. How old are you, Mrs. Sievert?"

"Thirty-one, well, I'll be thirty-two next month, I guess I should say I'm thirty-two to a doctor. But I tell everybody else I'm thirty-one. I'm not thirty-something yet!"

"And have you had any major health problems -- high blood pressure, diabetes, so forth?"

382

"No, nothing like that. My periods were pretty irregular until I started taking birth control pills."

"Any other symptoms? Chest pain? Abdominal pain? Fever? Pain anywhere?"

"No, just this breathing thing. Maybe some tightness in my chest."

"Has anything happened to upset you?"

"No, nothing in particular. Just, you know, the usual stresses."

"Sure?"

"Well, I mean, I knew he was going to leave sooner or later.

"He?"

"Well, my boyfriend. Up and left today, or I mean yesterday. Moved out. Not so much as a word of explanation. Said he'd had enough."

"And naturally that upset you."

"Not that much. He'd been saying he might leave for awhile now. Even kept playing that song about By the Time I Get to Phoenix. Played it over and over."

"Yes. Well, I don't think you have anything to worry about here. What you've described is the typical hyperventilation syndrome. You get a little nervous, or maybe have a bad dream. Then you unconsciously start overbreathing. Strangely, this makes you feel *more* short of breath. You have the sensation that the air won't get all the way to the bottom of your lungs. You blow off too much carbon dioxide from your system, and this makes your hands and feet start feeling numb, or as you say, tingly. The hands

383

and feet can even draw up -- we call this carpo-pedal spasm. You get dizzy, or spacy, feel like you're floating. Anybody can reproduce this just by hyperventilating. Somebody comes in the emergency clinic every day with this."

"But what causes it, Doctor?"

"Well, Helen, usually some emotional thing. You get anxious, the process starts, then you become alarmed by the symptoms, you hyperventilate more. A vicious cycle is underway. We see it all the time."

"What can I do?"

"It's simple. First, recognize that you're not dying, not even sick. Then get a paper bag, hold it tightly over your nose and mouth, and rebreathe. That is, in and out of the sack so that you keep breathing the same air for a while. Or just hold your breath. The carbon dioxide will build back up, the tingling and lightheadedness will go away. You'll feel better in no time."

"Oh, thanks, Doctor. I feel better already just talking to you."

"Maybe take a little tranquilizer or sedative. Do you have anything like that around?"

"I think there's some Donnatal in the cabinet from when I had stomach spasms."

"That's fine. Just take one of those." (I know this has a little phenobarbital in it.)

"And, Helen."

"Yes?"

"Think about what's been going on. See if you deal realistically with these things that have been happening. Ask

384

yourself, Are you worse off? Or better? Don't do that tonight, but tomorrow."

"Oh, OK. I'll -- do that. Thank you very much, Doctor."

I hang up the phone and roll back, flicking off the light in one motion. Wonder if Mary Alice woke up. Pretty good, the way I handled that. Helen will probably sleep well the rest of the night.

But will I?

Hyperventilation is, you see, a funny thing. I remember that guy last month who had it and turned out to have a heart attack. Ended up getting cathed and operated on for coronary disease. And that woman who developed it right after she delivered a baby -- turned out to have pulmonary emboli, innumerable clots to the lungs. Did OK after anticoagulation with heparin. And the lady who had an absolutely typical anxiety-hyperventilation episode but really had urinary tract infection, bacteremia (bacteria in the blood), and got really sick, took her a week to get over it on IV antibiotics in the hospital. Reminds me of that article in the *Archives* -- fifteen cases of hyperventilation which were really something else -- ruptured peptic ulcers, pneumothorax, etc.

I sit up on the edge of the bed. Maybe I better call Helen back. Here she is, apparently the first episode of this kind. Maybe it's the first sign of another disease process, something more serious. Just started on birth-control pills -- could she have developed phlebitis and pulmonary emboli herself? But what will I ask her or say to her? Will I tell her

385

to meet me at the emergency clinic? Examine her, get chest X-rays, urinalysis, blood work, chest film? Maybe even a lung scan? Total cost, about $1850? A hundred to one find nothing? Get her very upset? Will I see and do a detailed evaluation of this kind on every single case of hyperventilation? If I don't will I be doing a good, thorough job? If not, am I guilty of malpractice? Would a jury think so?

Or will I use my medical and common sense? Conclude that this is certainly a benign thing. Let her sleep. Know that if she's not OK she's intelligent enough to call me back? Ring her up in the early morning and make sure she's all right?

Yes, certainly. Fight off the evil humors of the night. Use daylight judgment. Roll back into bed and stare at the vaguely perceived off-white ceiling. Time to sleep.

At least for Mary Alice and Helen.

AGAIN THE DAWN

"NO MATTER WHERE YOU'VE ALWAYS BOUGHT YOUR GROCERIES YOU HAVEN'T SMART-SHOPPED UNTIL YOU'VE SHOPPED AT KIRBY'S . . ."

The snooze-button works, Thank God.

It's six a. m. I slept in an extra hour.

Bathrobe feels warm.

Coffee-water on.

Today's a running day.

Too tired.

Wonder how they're all doing.   Well, I'll see them soon enough.

But . . . I pick up the telephone.

"What's happening with Miss Rhonda this morning?"

"She's behaving pretty well.   Scheduled to go to the psych unit at 10 a. m.," Marie-Claire says.

"Thanks. I'll see her later."

"Fine. I'll tell her. She's --"

"What?"

"I don't know, still kind of mad."

"Good. That beats depressed."

"That's for sure."

I sip some coffee.   It's not bad.   My only cooking success.

"Bessie woke up and thought her right arm was paralyzed again, Dr. Galen," says Marlene. "'Course it made us worry about another transient ischemic attack." Marlene is from Alsace and in addition to being a hell of a nurse serves as my informal on-the-job French tutor.

"Uh-oh."

"But then it cleared up and now she says she slept on it wrong."

"Good. *Bon. C'est possible, certainement."*

"Oui. Mais je pense qu'elle ne sait pas."

"Trop rapidement, Marlene. Lentement, s'il vous plait, lentement.

"Oui. Je - pense - qu'elle - ne --"

"Right. I've got it, now. I agree that Bessie doesn't really know whether sleeping on it is the cause of the transient weakness or not. Let's make sure we get those vascular studies as early as possible this morning so we can see if she has any element of carotid stenosis --"

"Too fast, Doctor. Slowly, please, slowly."

The coffee must be working.

"OK, Marlene. Let's - make - sure - we - get - those - vascular --"

"Oui, oui, je comprend maintenant, je comprend."

"But I mean does Mr. Patton act *funny* in any way. Any peculiar statements or like that?"

"No," says Melissa. I don't know Melissa.

"But his blood sugar you say was 60?"

"At six a. m."

"And that's the lowest since we started treatment?"

"Yessir."

"Glucose still running?"

"Yessir."

"OK, sometimes it takes days to get over hypoglycemia caused by those pills. Let's just watch him and keep up his accuchecks."

"Yessir."

"The drug store hasn't called him again, have they?"

"Sir?"

"Never mind. Private joke. But not much of a joke."

"Oh."

"Tell you about it when I get there."

"Yessir."

I guess I still don't know Melissa.

The second cup of coffee is half regular and half decaf.

"She's capturing fine, Dr. Galen, according to CCU. Looks like she's totally pacemaker-dependent, though," Bob Seymour, 5 North nurse, says. I hear some noise, so it sounds as if Bob is standing in the nursing unit looking at the overnight report from the telemetry team on Mrs. Croft.

"Oh sure, she's been completely dependent on that thing for years. No pauses, though? Even when she moves around?"

"No. Clicking right along."

"Good. Dr. Platman and his team are going to put her through her paces this morning. Calisthenics and such."

"What?"

"Make sure the pacer doesn't flop around any more."

"Excuse me, but isn't she 82 years old?"

"About. Don't worry, they won't do aerobics."

"His 6 a. m. K hasn't been come back yet, it's only 6:30 now, Dr. Galen, but the 3 a. m. number was, let's see -- Randolph Brown -- it was 4.6."

"Great. Did you, I'm trying to think, call and tell me that earlier? I'm a little foggy this morning."

"No, sir, you left orders not to call if it was below 6."

"Oh. Right. How's he doing generally?"

"Well, vital signs stable. And he's in there making jokes."

"That's good. Last night he was making waves."

"So I hear."

PHOENIX RISING

"I know you probably have something else to do at 7 a.m. besides talk to me, Juanita," I say to the ICU-Blue head nurse.

"I'm happy to talk to you when there's good news."

"Really? About Sydney?"

"Yes. Urinary output has jumped up to 600 cc in the last 8 hours."

"Great."

"Oxygen saturation has improved. We've cut the flow and we've even been able to reduce the end-expiratory pressure on the ventilator."

"Terrific."

"And, this isn't for sure yet, but I think it's a change."

"What's that?"

"When we turn the Versed drip down, he starts moving around and groaning. Makes purposeful movements."

"That's all wonderful, Juanita. Would you like to come and work for me?"

"What's the weekend schedule?"

"Probably better than the job you have. Has the family heard about the improvements?"

"Sure, I let them know. They're cheering. I told them not to get too excited yet."

"Good work. There's one other person who would love to know all this."

"Oh, yes. Dr. Jeffrey Owens. I have a page in to him. He was looking bad yesterday, almost as bad as the patient."

"But when you tell him, he'll get well quick. Quicker than Sydney."

"Renal Transplant Unit. This is Connie."

"Dr. Galen, Connie." I find I don't have the courage to ask if the cross-match was OK. Beating around the bush is easier.

"When do you think they'll take Karen Coberley down? I wanted to stick my head in." I'm holding my breath.

"Oh, she's long gone. They did her about 4 a. m. She's in ICU Blue already. A three-antigen match, you know, cross-match negative. They said everything went great. Put out urine on the table. She has a cheering section down in the waiting room, all her friends and half the lawyers in town."

I finally exhale. "Making sure we don't screw up, huh?"

Connie chuckles. "I don't know. Actually, they all seemed to be more like -- *praying*."

"Lawyers? Praying?"

"Yessir. You have to realize, Dr. Galen, this transplantation thing is a modern miracle."

"You've convinced me, Connie. Thanks."

And thanks, big thanks, to the One they were praying to.

     I realize full well the nurses have something else to do besides talk to a curious physician at dawn. They have to "do report" -- exchange information on the patients, get the medication cart ready for a. m. rounds, check vital signs, dressings, weigh patients, change beds, and bathe bed patients. Key in all that stuff on the computer. Also look good when the unit supervisor walks through. To say nothing of catch up on last night's social happenings.

     Too bad, but I just can't wait.

     "Is this CCU?"

     "Yes, this is Madison."

     "Madison, this is Dr. Galen. Dr. Galen, Jr., is taking care of him, but I was just wondering about Henry Adams. Are you looking after him?"

     "Oh, yes. Had some ventricular ectopy during the night with a little coupling but no more v. tach or anything like that. On a beta-blocker, lidocaine drip still. No pain. Looks pretty good."

     "Are the cardiologists planning anything?"

     "They're talking about cath, maybe angioplasty later this morning, but I don't think they've got a time yet."

     "How's he taking all this?'

     "How do you mean?"

     "I mean, is he upset and agitated?"

     "Seems pretty calm to me. Gave him a little Valium at about 3 a. m."

392

"How's his wife holding up?"

"OK, I guess. She stayed all night."

"I was busy last night, never got to see her, only talked on the phone."

"The cardiologist talked to her, and don't worry, Dr. Johnny held her hand until about five a. m."

"Dr. Johnny?"

"Dr. Galen, Jr."

"Does he know he's Dr. Johnny?"

"I think so." Madison laughs. "I think he likes that better than what we were calling him."

"Which was?"

"Dr. Boy."

"How's Cora Jones acting this morning, Della?"

"She's just fine. We took her restraints off last night. She's up in a chair already, eating. The printout hasn't come back, but I can get the 6 a. m. lab on the computer. Just a minute."

"Don't spend your time doing that, I'll check by in a little while."

"No, that's OK, this new computer is great. If I can just get into the dam-- dern thing at all. Excuse me."

There is a moment of silence.

"Sodium 129. I know that's the main one you were interested in."

"Right."

"SAD -- what was it Juanita said this was?"

"SIADH."

"And what does it mean?"

"Get Juanita to tell you. She should be an expert by now. She's probably deep into the library Medline system as we speak, of course."

"Sure. If that's a new type of mattress."

"Well, she was very interested in this. Probably dreaming about serum sodiums right now."

"Probably. I'll ask her to do an in-service on it."

"When she wakes up."

"Right."

The BMW cranks right up this time. Temperature's already 58.

Nice to know everybody's doing well, particularly after spending all night down there. Almost worth it.

Definitely worth it.

Seems as if I forgot to check on somebody, though. Oh well, it'll come to me.

EMERGENCY - CALL 350-3346 - NURSE GLENDA - PATIENT THOMAS HOPPER - HEMORRHAGING. EMERGENCY. PLEASE CONFIRM WITH ANSWERING SERVICE - EMERGENCY

It's come to me, all right. Thomas -- Satchmo -- bleeding somewhere. I'll go straight to intensive care. The BMW is beginning to hum now.

ROGER ELDER   - 321- 1874 - REPORTS LAXATIVE TOO EFFECTIVE

394

Sandra can talk to Mr. Elder. I'll take care of Satchmo. And Jimmy Treadway. Then the other hospital patients. Then the office patients. Then the telephone.

Then, late in the afternoon, as the bright October sun spreads into a thousand wispy rays across the sky before it melts into the horizon, there will be a big change in the nature of the day.

I won't be on call anymore. For a while.

And I can sleep.

AFTERWORD

You have perhaps wondered if Dr John Galen's strenuous schedule is practical, or if it would even last in our contemporary leisure society.

The answer is no.

You see, the urban primary care physician in 2005 America, such as the internist or family physician, no longer works 70-80 hours per week, with 2 or 3 on-calls per week. He sees patients for an average of 35 hours, with little or no on-call. He either finishes up his shift in the outpatient clinic and goes home, or he is a hospitalist, doing work only in the inpatient setting . . . 35 hours either way.

The pre-med students are in sync with this concept; candidates will boldly tell members of an admissions committee that they "want a life" (translation: off at 5 o'clock). New internists just out of training will apply only for jobs with salaries, no overhead, and fixed hours.

Some say this leads to greater medical and cost-efficiency. Others complain that the doctor should not abandon his regular patient at the moment of her greatest need – when hospitalization is necessary, or at night when that emergency surfaces.

Earlier concerns about the "doctor glut" have disappeared -- not because of shrinkage of physician number but by a reduction in physician-hours. It would now take two Dr. Galens to do the job described in this book.

The other change is a result of managed care measures imposed by Medicare and the insurance companies, each encouraging the other. Reduction of reimbursement and expansion of paperwork requirements would have fiscally disenfranchised the profession had not the doctors been reasonably clever. You're giving us half the pay? Heck, we'll double the number of patients. The patient load in the office has increased from about 13 a day per internist in 1984 to about 25 in 2004. Do the math: that's half as much time with each patient. Half as much history. Half as much physical. Half as much bonding.

Time will tell how this all comes out. But John Galen sure had a good time.